Francis J Browne
(1879–1963)

A Biography

Francis J Browne
(1879–1963)
A Biography

Herbert E Reiss

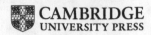

Shaftesbury Road, Cambridge CB2 8EA, United Kingdom

One Liberty Plaza, 20th Floor, New York, NY 10006, USA

477 Williamstown Road, Port Melbourne, VIC 3207, Australia

314–321, 3rd Floor, Plot 3, Splendor Forum, Jasola District Centre, New Delhi – 110025, India

103 Penang Road, #05–06/07, Visioncrest Commercial, Singapore 238467

Cambridge University Press is part of Cambridge University Press & Assessment,
a department of the University of Cambridge.

We share the University's mission to contribute to society through the pursuit of
education, learning and research at the highest international levels of excellence.

www.cambridge.org
Information on this title: www.cambridge.org/9781904752103

A catalogue record for this publication is available from the British Library

ISBN   978-1-904-75210-3   Hardback

Published by the RCOG Press at the
Royal College of Obstetricians and Gynaecologists
27 Sussex Place, Regent's Park
London NW1 4RG

Registered Charity No. 213280

Cover image: FJ Browne; photograph held in the Archives of the Royal Australian and
New Zealand College of Obstetricians and Gynaecologists

RCOG Press Editor: Elisabeth Rees-Evans
Index: Liza Furnival, Medical Indexing Ltd
Design & typesetting: Karl Harrington, FiSH Books

To those who have taught
me and to those I have taught

Herbert E Reiss
11 February 2005

Contents

Illustrations

Foreword

Thomas Carlyle wrote 'biography is the most universally pleasant, the most universally profitable of all reading'. Having just read this biography of FJ Browne by Herbert Reiss, I am in total agreement. FJ's time was not so long ago yet how different were people's lives, their social circumstances, the clinical and academic environment. What an extraordinary career FJ had. The fourth of eight children of a County Donegal farmer; rejected by the Civil Service; joined and then left the Irish Guards; studied medicine in Aberdeen; spent thirteen years in general practice in a Welsh mining town; took up obstetrics at the age of 39 and worked for Ballantyne in Edinburgh; was appointed to the first chair in obstetrics and gynaecology in London in 1926 at UCH; and after retirement in 1946, began a new life in Australia in 1951. I hope I have succeeded in whetting your appetite. Getting inside this man and learning about his life and times and achievements has been fascinating. In a deft and vivid portrait, Herbert Reiss has done this great man justice and in so doing, has enriched us.

Charles Rodeck

Preface and acknowledgements

In 1946 I attended Professor FJ Browne's last lecture before his retirement from the Chair of Obstetrics and Gynaecology at University College Hospital, London. Although I was only in my first year as a clinical student, and not yet doing obstetrics, his fame was so great that this was an occasion not to be missed. (Later I was taught by his former assistants: Gladys Dodds, Tim Flew, Fouracre Barnes and Dame Josephine Barnes, to all of whom I owe sincere gratitude.)

FJ (as he was universally known) was tall, almost gaunt, slightly stooped, with receding silver-grey hair, a high forehead, prominent nose, slightly bulging eyes and a black moustache. He spoke with a soft Irish accent. He was wearing a long white coat. The lecture theatre was packed. He lectured, without notes, on postpartum haemorrhage. The subject was covered in a masterly manner. I still remember its substance. What is more important is the way in which he was communicating directly with his audience, leaning over the podium, looking at them as he addressed them and speaking to them, not at them. Here was a real teacher.

Francis James Browne (1879–1963) was born in Ireland. He qualified in medicine in Scotland in 1906 and worked as a general practitioner in Wales until 1919 when he became assistant to Dr JW Ballantyne in Edinburgh. In 1926 he was appointed Professor of Obstetrics and Gynaecology at University College Hospital, London. After his retirement and the death of his first wife, he remarried in 1951 and settled in Sydney, Australia where he died in 1963. He became the foremost obstetrician of his day and the founder of modern antenatal care.

His book *Antenatal and Postnatal Care* became the best of its kind and a bible to many generations of medical students and junior obstetricians. Our ideal was to follow the high standards of observation, manual dexterity and note keeping he had set.

For someone who not only made a major contribution to his field, but also enjoyed the company of so many friends and colleagues, it is remarkable how little is known of his personal life. Tracing his history has been a great adventure. In this I have been most ably assisted by his grandsons, Geoffrey Browne and David Hurford, and by the nephew of his second wife, Chris Cuthbert. Others whose assistance I was glad to accept include: in Ireland, May McClintock, local historian, and Alan Roberts of Foyle College Old Boys' Association; in Scotland, A Adam of the Aberdeen Medico-Chirurgical Society, Steve Kerr, assistant librarian of the Royal College of Surgeons, Edinburgh, and Iain Milne, librarian of the Royal College of Physicians Edinburgh; in Wales, Hugh Watkins of Abertillery Library, Keith Thomas, Don Bearcroft and Frances Younson; in England, Sir John Peel, Sir Stanley Simmons, TLT Lewis (deceased), Peter Fell, Professor Norman Morris, Elliot Philipp, Professor Charles Rodeck, Patricia Want, Germaine Greer, Ashley Ashford-Brown, David Boyle, convenor of the Gynaecological Visiting Society, John Wells, Cambridge University Library, Neena Lubotacky and Julia Reiss; in Australia, Ian Cope (deceased), Rosalind Winspear of the Royal Australian and New Zealand College of Obstetricians and Gynaecologists, Francis Reiss and Mark Reiss.

Miss Patricia Want, former Head of the Markland Library and Information Services at the Royal College of Obstetricians and Gynaecologists has compiled an excellent bibliography, without which this book would be the poorer.

Many more helped and failure to record all their names is no reflection on the role they played in the compilation of this story. Professors Peter Curzen and Michael Reiss kindly read the drafts and made many corrections and suggestions. To all of them I am deeply grateful. Interpretation of their information and any opinions expressed are entirely my own responsibility.

Herbert E Reiss

Chapter One
From Tullybogly to Aberdeen

Francis James Browne was born in Ireland at Tullybogly, County Donegal, on 1 October 1879. His paternal grandparents, Adam (1809–1865) and Rebecca (1823–1888) Browne were farmers at Tullybogly, as were his parents, William (1854–1944) and Sarah Jane (née Galbraith, 1853–1933) Browne.

Tullybogly is about three miles east of the nearest village, Manorcunningham, eight miles east of Letterkenny and no more than 25 miles from Londonderry. It consists of three cottages with outbuildings, stables and cowsheds, and nestles in the green, gently undulating lowlands of County Donegal, not far from the shores of the beautiful Lough Swilly. It is too small to be called a village and the nearest church, shop and public house are at Manorcunningham. It is reached, with some effort, by country lanes which get ever narrower and more muddy. Signposts are few and getting there is difficult without a good sense of direction. The soil is rich, dark, productive and well watered, ideal for raising sheep and cattle, and growing corn, flax and potatoes. Manorcunningham is named after its first proprietor, James Cunningham, who in the 16th century erected the original castle and the surrounding villages. It has both a Roman Catholic church and a Presbyterian meeting house.

The house in which FJ was born – most deliveries took place at home in those days – has been rebuilt with the addition of a second storey, but is still a modest farm cottage with small rooms. It is difficult to see how it could accommodate a large

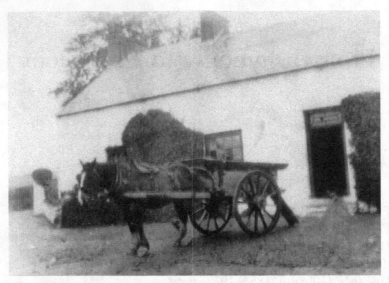
A faded image of Tullybogly, as it was in FJ's time

family. There is a small yard and garden and splendid views over the fields alive with the sheep, cattle and crops. At some stage FJ's father, William, bought the farm next door. After the death of William's wife, Sarah, one of their sons, Johnny, an older brother of FJ's, returned from New Zealand where he was a dairy farmer, to look after his old father and the farm. After Johnny's death, in 1953, the house was sold to the father of the present owners, Mr and Mrs McNaught, whilst the next door house was sold to Mr and Mrs McLean who still live there. Mrs McLean remembers William Browne well and knew most of his children.

William and Sarah Browne had eight children of whom FJ was the fourth. He was known throughout his life as FJ to most people but his many nephews and nieces called him Uncle Frank. His was a happy childhood and, as in almost any large family, his early upbringing was as much by his siblings as by his very busy father and mother.

His oldest brother, William Henry, an engineer, went to live in Renfrew, outside Glasgow. There he had two daughters and a son, also called William, who married Kathleen Ashford Collins and changed his name to Ashford-Brown (dropping the 'e'). At the age of 17 William had entered Glasgow University. He was too young for admission to the medical course and so, on Uncle Frank's advice, took a BSc degree before embarking on medicine. He wrote a small autobiography entitled *Cold Hands: the Memoirs of a Scottish GP* published in 1997. In it he describes his grandfather, William (FJ's father), as being 'very tall, straight backed, and bearded with grey eyes which always seemed to be looking into the distance and he seemed rather impeccably dressed for a farmer. He went everywhere by horse, a high spirited Arab, and trap'. FJ inherited some of these traits from his father – he too was tall and slim, not bearded but with a black moustache. In later years he became somewhat stooped and this is how his grandson Geoffrey remembers him. Dr Ashford Brown also remembers his grandmother, FJ's mother, Sarah,

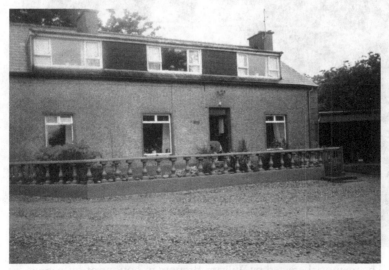

The house where Francis was born

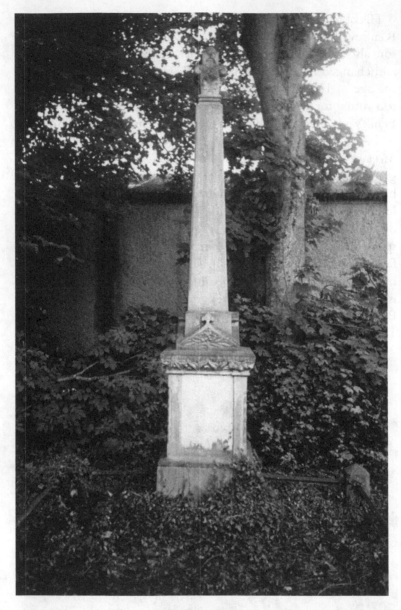

The memorial erected by William Browne in honour of his parents,
in the Anglican churchyard at Manorcunningham

whom he describes as 'a quiet little woman who always wore a white shawl. She was a wonderful cook and invariably had meals ready regularly at 8 am, 12 noon, 4 pm and 8 pm'.

Of FJ's other siblings, two, Sam and John, emigrated to the Antipodes, although John returned as described above. Matilda (Aunt Tilly) became a hospital matron; her fiancé died in the post-war influenza epidemic and she never married. Sadie, also a nurse, died unmarried in 1946. Elizabeth married William Wallace who owned a store in Manorcunningham and they had twin sons, Gerald and Ernest, who are alive and remember Uncle Frank well. Ruby died in 1900, ten years old, of tuberculosis.

In the Anglican churchyard in Manorcunningham there is a memorial erected by William Browne in honour of his parents, Adam and Rebecca. It is a large, impressive monument, situated at the far left-hand boundary of the churchyard, after one has gone along rows of old graves with their weathered and often leaning tombstones. The grave, as revealed by inscriptions, also contains the remains of William's wife, Sarah (1853–1933) and two of their daughters, Ruby who died in 1900 and Sadie who died in 1948, as well as his own remains following his death in 1944.

The first school FJ attended was the Balleighan National Primary School, about three miles from Tullybogly, on the east shore of Lough Swilly. The school no longer exists, but the house remains, not far from the birthplace of FJ's wife at Balleighan and near the ruins of a lovely 11th-century friary on the shore of the Lough. From the Balleighan National Primary School at the age of 12 or 13, FJ proceeded to the Raphoe Royal School, about seven miles from Tullybogly. The school had been re-opened in 1892 as a Protestant institution and at first had 20 pupils, both boys and girls. By 1894 this number had increased to 38 and reached 73 in 1898, mainly day pupils. FJ's father gave him a pony and trap for the journey.

FJ entered Foyle College in Londonderry on 3 September 1896, a few days before his 17th birthday and stayed there for the next five years until 1901. Foyle College was the successor to the

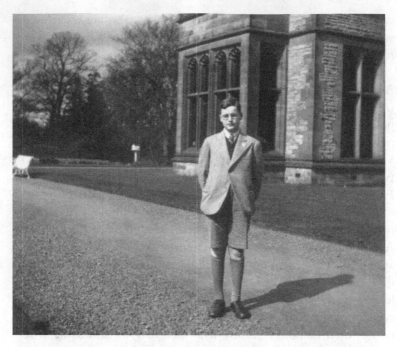

The young Francis at Foyle College, Londonderry

Derry Free Grammar School, founded in 1617, and amalgamated with the Londonderry Academical Institution in 1896. The old college was housed at that time in a commandingly situated building overlooking the Foyle river. It had an impressive staff which included four Cambridge MAs, two of them Wranglers, a gold medallist from Trinity College Dublin, two graduates from London University and others from leading English and Irish universities. This was the quality of the staff whilst FJ was at school there. There was a classical side for boys preparing to enter universities and a modern side for those preparing for the Civil Service and commercial pursuits. The college rightly had the reputation of being one of the best schools in Ireland. It was moved to a new site in 1967 and the old building is now the Londonderry Arts Centre. FJ's second wife, Grace, presented furnishings and a photograph of FJ which are now in the boardroom of the new school with a plaque which reads as follows:

> The panelling and furnishing of this room were provided by Dr Grace Browne in memory of her husband, Professor FJ Browne, MD, DSc, FRCSE, FRCOG, at Foyle College 1896–1901.

FJ attended Foyle College as a day boy and made the daily journeys by the Lough Swilly Railway. The journey from Manorcunningham to Derry took about one and a half hours – a demanding undertaking twice a day. Through lack of time, this meant that he was not able to join any of the school teams for organised games. FJ was President of the college's Old Boys' Association in 1946/47 and chaired in Derry the first dinner of the association after the war. To mark the occasion, he endowed a Memorial Prize for literature in his name: he himself was very fond of poetry and particularly of Shakespeare. The prize is still awarded annually, but now for music. It is of interest to note that a friend of his, Charles Macafee,[1] also attended Foyle College and was President of the Association 1964–1965.

FJ left school, 22 years old and restless like any young man of that age. There was much indecision about his future. The prospect of farming at Tullybogly did not attract him. He passed the Civil Service entry examinations, but was rejected at interview; according to one story because his hair and eyebrows were singed and hands blackened after fighting a fire at his father's farm the night before. He joined the Irish Guards in London but did not find army life to his satisfaction and was 'bought out'. One wonders who raised the necessary money. He returned to the family home, but soon ran away to work as a railway porter in Glasgow. These must have been brief episodes because in the autumn of 1901, the same year he left school, he entered Aberdeen University to study medicine. The usual choice of medical schools for those living in the region would have been Queen's College Belfast, Trinity College Dublin or Edinburgh, but, according to Gerald Wallace, Aberdeen offered the cheapest fees and lodgings. Even so, FJ had to borrow money and live on a diet mainly of porridge. The loans were eventually repaid after qualification and the financial situation as a student slightly improved when in 1902 FJ was awarded the Thompson Bursary for medical students entering their second year. This consisted of £20 per year for three years and was awarded by competition. He had lodgings at 42 Sunnybank Place and joined the University Company of the Royal Army Medical Corps. As a student, he was medallist in physics, medical jurisprudence and public health He qualified MB ChB, passing his finals in 1906 'with highest honours' and distinctions in pathology, medical jurisprudence and public health. The telegram he sent his parents reads: 'Results out. Passed with distinction'.

Note

1   Macafee became Professor of Obstetrics and Gynaecology in Belfast. He is particularly known for his classification of antepartum haemorrhage and of degrees of placenta praevia. In 1928 he invited FJ to become Examiner in Midwifery in the Belfast Final Examinations – a welcome opportunity for FJ to visit his home and family.

Chapter Two

The Abertillery years
1906–1919

A newly qualified doctor has a choice of 30 to 40 different careers. Most of them involve specialising, which implies long periods of time for, in those days, negligible remuneration. FJ, having attained distinctions in most subjects in his final examination, could certainly have achieved a resident appointment at his teaching hospital: a sure first step on the career ladder. Instead, in 1906, immediately after qualifying, he settled in Abertillery, a small mining town in South Wales. He was keen to get started in the practice of medicine as quickly as possible and. intent on paying off his debts so that he could get married. In those days practices had to be bought, for which he did not have the capital, or involved 'putting up a plate' and waiting for patients, for which he did not have time. He opted therefore for a salaried post in a practice attached to a colliery. Abertillery at that time would have been described, in modern parlance, as an economically and socially deprived area. Sited in the steep hills and deep valleys of Monmouthshire, it had existed as a small settlement since prehistoric and Roman times. There are remains of medieval barns and dwellings and an ancient stone bridge at the junction of the Tyleri and Ebbw Fach rivers.

The beautiful, heavily wooded district was spoiled by the ravages of the Industrial Revolution. The Abertillery tin works were opened in 1846 and the first mine shafts sunk in 1850. Further pits were opened in the next decade. By the time FJ came, there were ten tin works with over 400 workers and at

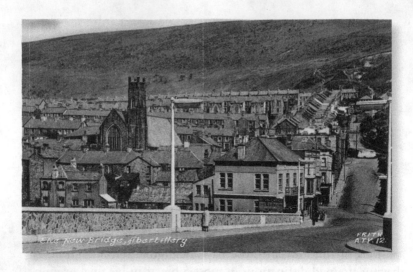

A view of Abertillery captured in an old postcard

least six collieries, employing several thousands of miners. Iron foundries were started in the 1860s with plants to produce steel. With the production of coal, tin, iron and steel, modern methods of transport were needed to replace mules and horse-drawn barges. Roads, railways and canals were built. Within a short time, the local population increased sharply from the 800-odd inhabitants before the 19th century. Factories, foundries, high chimneys and pitheads dominated the scene, and new streets with workers' houses ran up and down the narrow valleys. Employment, especially in the mines, was hazardous with a high incidence of accidents and explosions, causing many deaths. Work was hard, wages were low, with workers having to buy their own tools, and conditions were terrible with dirt, dust, static water, rats, poor ventilation and roof falls. The frequent deaths of miners caused much distress among relatives and comrades. Sickness and deaths from cholera and dysentery were frequent. At the same time, the number of births was soaring owing to the influx of more workers, with their number reaching nearly 20,000.

Such was the scene which greeted FJ as a newly qualified and inexperienced doctor. There were few doctors in the town and they were mostly attached to a company or colliery. FJ started work immediately at the Arrael Griffin (Six Bells) colliery. These were founded in 1891; the number of miners in 1913 was 1,884 with an output of about 450,000 tons of coal a year. An explosion at the Six Bells colliery in 1960 killed 45 men. A

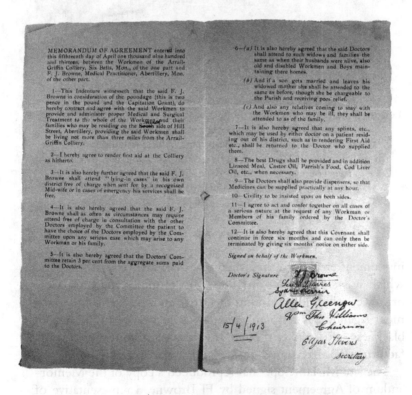

The memorandum of agreement signed by FJ Browne
and the Arrael Griffin (Six Bells) colliery

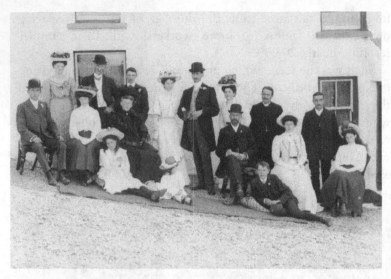

The Gallaugher family at Greenbank, Donegal, on the occasion of
the marriage of Mary to Francis Browne.
Left to right: (back row) a wedding guest, Mr Browne, John Browne,
Mary (Minnie) Gallaugher, Francis (Frank) Browne,
Jeannie Gallaugher, the Minister, Willie Gallaugher;
(front row, seated) John Gallaugher, Sadie Browne, Mrs Browne,
two young guests, John Gallaugher, Neil McCord
(sitting on the ground), Tilly Browne, Lizzie Browne

monument erected to their memory marks the site of the mine
which was closed down in 1986. All the mines and most factories were shut down around this time and the Welsh Development Agency has restored greenness and beauty to an area of
blackness and smoke, though the loss of mining and manu-
facturing jobs has caused distress and social upheaval.

The late Mr Ian Cope[1] has reproduced a copy of the Memorandum of Agreement signed by FJ Browne, a representative of
the workers and the company secretary, dated 15 April 1913. The
original is now in the archives of the Royal Australian and New

Zealand College of Obstetricians and Gynaecologists. In this it is stipulated that, in return for a capitation fee, he, in association with other doctors employed by the Committee, assumed medical and surgical care of the workmen and their families (if they lived within three miles of the colliery), rendered first aid, attended 'lying-in cases' and provided medical care to widows and their families and to disabled workers. The best drugs and food supplements were to be provided and 'civility was to be insisted upon on both sides'. There is no doubt that this work represented a large portion of his practice. The rising birth rate and the custom of having babies at home meant that a great deal of the general practitioner's workload in those days consisted of midwifery. Abnormalities such as haemorrhage, eclampsia,

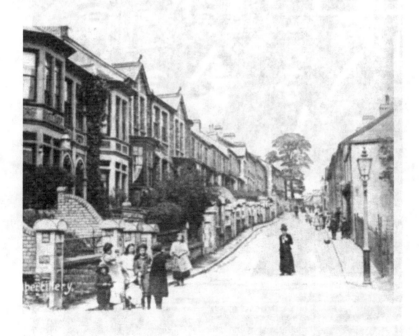

Alma Street, Abertillery; FJ and Minnie lived at number 35
(courtesy of Mr Keith Thomas)

breech presentation or transverse lie of the fetus were managed in the patient's own home by the attending general practitioner. FJ thus acquired extensive experience in midwifery which stood him in good stead in later job applications. Having to climb the steep streets of the town, with large distances to cover and a heavy medical bag to carry, made it essential for FJ to acquire a pony and trap as means of transport.

The years in Abertillery were eventful. On 6 August 1908 he married Mary (1884–1948), usually known as Minnie, daughter of John Gallaugher, at Manorcunningham. The house in which Minnie was born is a large farmhouse at Balleighan, not far from

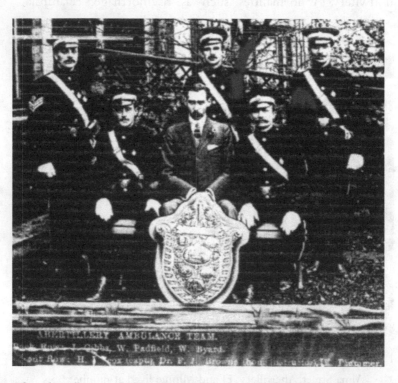

The Abertillery Ambulance Team with the Martin Shield, which they won on a regular basis (courtesy of Mr Keith Thomas)

Manorcunningham. There are beautiful gardens and fields sloping down to Lough Swilly. Isolated in a superb position, it has been rebuilt and modernised and is now owned by Mr and Mrs Brendon McLaughlin. It is larger and more prosperous-looking than FJ's own birthplace. Sheep and cattle graze on the slopes where rabbits, foxes and badgers roam and dolphins, seals and otters are seen in the Lough. There are extensive outbuildings, cattle sheds and a paddock for the horses.

FJ brought Minnie to Abertillery where they acquired a house at 35 Alma Street. This was a modest residence with two rooms per floor, on a steep street facing open land. It was here that their first two children were born, Olive in 1909 and John McClure in 1912.

Even with a large and busy practice, FJ found time to act as temporary medical officer of health and public vaccinator for Abertillery District. Universal vaccination was then customary as smallpox was still widespread. He became medical officer of the St John Ambulance team; the team won the Martin Shield in the years 1911, 1912, 1915 and 1919.

In addition to all these tasks, FJ took, and passed in 1914, the Fellowship examination of the Edinburgh Royal College of Surgeons. The regulations for that year required that 'Every candidate shall pass (a) an examination on the principles and practice of surgery, including surgical anatomy, (b) clinical surgery and (c) one optional subject'. FJ took advanced midwifery with obstetric surgery as his optional. The examination consisted of written, oral and clinical or practical work. The Fellowship was awarded by ballot of the examiners. Three-fourths of the votes was required to entitle the candidate to be admitted and the number of those voting was not less than twenty. This was an unusual qualification for a general practitioner to acquire. Aspiring surgeons with the Fellowship who did not make the grade to become consultants or needed to start earning a reasonable living often entered general practice − but the opposite pathway was highly unusual. It must have required a tremendous amount of hard work for someone based in

University of Aberdeen.

This is to Certify that on the occasion of his being admitted by this University to the Degree of Doctor of Medicine, Francis James Browne was awarded Highest Honours for the Thesis submitted by him.

George Adam Smith
Principal

F. Sherman. M.D.
Dean of Medical Faculty

D.R. Thom
Secretary.

11ᵗʰ July, 1919.

FJ Browne's MD certificate from the University of Aberdeen
(courtesy of the Dean)

general practice instead of a hospital environment to pass such an examination and further proof of FJ's ambition and determination.

In the World War, in September 1915 FJ volunteered for service with the forces and joined up as a lieutenant in the Royal Army Medical Corps. He served mainly as medical officer on the British Hospital Ship *St George*. Their main task was the evacuation of wounded personnel from France. However, it proved impossible to find a locum tenens to carry on his practice and as the area was of industrial importance, the Secretary of the British Medical Association and the local Member of Parliament requested his return to Abertillery on account of the shortage of local doctors. Reluctantly he resigned his commission in 1916. He volunteered again to rejoin the RAMC in August 1916 and May 1917, but on both occasions was refused a commission by the War Office, as a result of the intervention of the Central War Emergency Committee of the British Medical Association. He therefore returned to his practice and also carried on the work of another, and for part of the time of two other, local medical men. In addition to all this, at this time he became a school medical officer.

Even this was not enough. The obstetric experience in Abertillery had triggered a lasting interest in the subject and gradually led to the desire to specialise in this branch of medicine. He had attended postgraduate courses in London (1911) and Edinburgh (1912 and 1913) and in 1918 took time off his practice to do a 3-month resident post at the Edinburgh Royal Infirmary. Usually such posts are held by much younger doctors. FJ was now a 39-year-old married man. To take such a post, working with junior colleagues, and having to cope with numerous night calls, little sleep and poor accommodation is a demanding undertaking for the more mature doctor.

During this residency, he had a patient with a hydatidiform mole and lutein cysts of the ovary. This is a potentially serious abnormality of the placenta, which may cause heavy bleeding in early pregnancy and may proceed to form a malignant tumour of the uterus. In a mole, the chorionic villi swell and are distended with fluid, and the placenta resembles a bunch of grapes. Usually there is no fetus. FJ made a detailed pathological and histological study of the specimen uterus and placenta and of the changes in the ovaries. He submitted these studies in 1919 as a thesis for the Aberdeen MD degree, entitled 'A contribution to the study of hydatidiform mole with special reference to its association with lutein cysts in the ovary'. The role of lutein cysts in the ovary to the mole itself had long been a subject of dispute. FJ believed that vascular degeneration in the ovary led to the pathological changes he had studied. The concept of the ovarian changes being of primary importance, causing the placental changes, is not in accord with present-day thinking. But Browne also speculated that there might be an antenatal conceptual pathology for these changes 'in which the male must for the first time be thought to bear his due responsibility'. This concept, that the male might be involved, anticipated the present-day findings that there are genetic abnormalities involved in the aetiology of hydatidiform mole, such as triploidy with one maternal and two paternal sets of chromosomes or the fertilisation of an egg with a degenerated nucleus by an abnormal sperm. He was awarded the degree 'with highest honours'.

Studies such as these are not usually undertaken by general practitioners. They are clear evidence not only of an enquiring mind's intelligence and application, but also of FJ's ultimate ambition to devote himself entirely to the practice of obstetrics and gynaecology.

Note

1 *Australian and New Zealand Journal of Obstetrics and Gynaecology* 1988;28:85–89.

Chapter Three
Edinburgh 1919–1926

Following his short period as a gynaecological resident in Edinburgh, FJ wrote on 18 November 1918 to Dr John Ballantyne, one of the teachers on the postgraduate courses he had attended, applying for the post of obstetric resident at the Simpson Memorial Hospital.

Ballantyne (1861–1923) was the outstanding pioneer of antenatal care. Originally trained as a pathologist, he had chosen as a subject for his Edinburgh MD thesis 'Some anatomical and pathological conditions of the new-born infant in relation to obstetrics'. For this he was awarded a gold medal. His aim and hope was to reduce the incidence of stillbirths and congenital fetal abnormalities by better antenatal care of the pregnant woman. He considered that maternal consumption of alcohol, nicotine and lead, and infections such as syphilis and tuberculosis were significant hazards for the fetus and should be treated during the pregnancy. He was a man of great vision and soon was appointed lecturer in antenatal pathology and teratology, later becoming assistant physician and in 1904 chief physician at the Edinburgh Royal Infirmary. He introduced the concept that sick pregnant women should be looked after by obstetricians rather than by general physicians. Before this time the obstetrician usually saw his patient for the first time in advanced labour and then only if called in by the attending midwife, for delay in labour, malpresentations or haemorrhage.

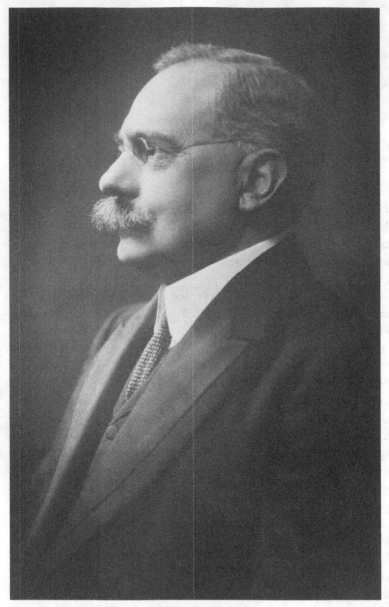

John Ballantyne

Ballantyne wrote widely on antenatal diagnosis and thera-
peutics and called for the establishment of 'pre-maternity hospitals' where obstetricians could care for pregnant women and
study the physiology of normal and abnormal pregnancy. As a
result of his pleas, the first antenatal bed in the world was
endowed at the Edinburgh Royal Infirmary in 1901 by the
generous gift of £1,000 from Dr Freeland Barbour, consultant
at the infirmary and past president of the Edinburgh Obstetrical
Society. Ballantyne was put in charge of it. With the aid of Dr
Haig Ferguson, a refuge for unmarried women was established
and this became the precursor of antenatal clinics throughout
the world. This afforded an opportunity for patients to rest, be
fed adequately and have their anaemia corrected. It led to the
introduction of external cephalic version to convert a breech to
a cephalic presentation. It also provided the first opportunity for
the study of abnormalities in pregnancy, such as eclampsia, hyperemesis, jaundice, hydramnios, abortion and hydatidiform mole.
A scholar by nature, Ballantyne wrote numerous books and very
many articles on obstetric and gynaecological subjects and was
regarded as one of the foremost teachers in Edinburgh at that
time.

The Simpson Memorial Hospital, the obstetric department of
the Edinburgh Royal Infirmary, was named after Sir James Young
Simpson (1811–1870), the great Edinburgh obstetrician and
gynaecologist. One of Simpson's many achievements and invent-
ions was the introduction, in 1847, of chloroform for inhalation
anaesthesia at delivery. The 'old' Simpson Hospital was first
opened in 1879 and had 65 beds. In 1910, there were 616
deliveries in hospital, whilst there were 1,327 district deliveries.
The hospital closed in 1939 when a new department, the
Simpson Memorial Pavilion, was opened with 126 beds.

FJ by now had his eye on a consultant appointment in his
chosen subject in South Wales.[1] He saw little prospect of obtaining such a post without further resident hospital experience and
wrote to Ballantyne in this connection. Much to his surprise,
Ballantyne replied offering him a post as his assistant. FJ wanted

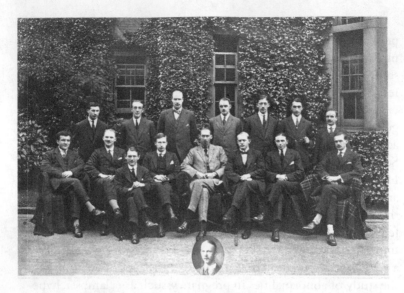

Residents at the Royal Infirmary of Edinburgh, 1918

to accept this opportunity more than anything else, but there was one major problem: the post carried a salary of only £400 per annum. He was married and had, by this time, two young children to bring up and educate and could ill afford to give up a relatively lucrative practice in Abertillery. Faced with such a dilemma, and having to make the most momentous decision of his professional life, he had a sleepless night and a tortured day. Finally he went into the small post office in Lauriston Place, very near the 'old Simpson' and sent a telegram to Mary. As told by Chassar Moir (GVS oration), 'anxious hours followed. Again and again he returned expectantly and again and again he left disappointed. But at last an answer arrived. The telegram from his wife contained only one word: 'ACCEPT'.

The family moved into 54 Northumberland Street, north of Princes Street and within walking distance of Lauriston Place, the site of the Royal Infirmary and Simpson Memorial Hospital. His official status was research pathologist with additional duties as assistant in the antenatal and VD departments. Ballantyne, his chief, guided and advised FJ and became a strongly formative influence on his development. He set an example FJ aspired to follow. It is significant that when he later wrote his book *Antenatal and Postnatal Care*, he dedicated it to Ballantyne.

FJ's post in Edinburgh afforded him a period of enormous activity in clinical medicine and, for the first time in his life, introduced him to the field of research. FJ was also appointed clinical tutor at the Royal Infirmary and started teaching both undergraduates and postgraduates, thus supplementing his meagre salary. His classes soon became highly popular and well attended.

His first major publication[2] was on anencephaly, a major fetal abnormality in which the vault of the skull and brain are grossly underdeveloped and which invariably leads to neonatal death. Browne's detailed and scholarly paper describes the anatomical and pathological features of this condition which are usually correlated with the absence of the pituitary gland. Other publications followed: on syphilis and the Wassermann reaction in pregnancy; on abnormalities of the umbilical cord which may cause antenatal death of the fetus; on post-maturity; and on causes, pathology and prevention of abortions and stillbirths. At the BMA Annual Meeting in Glasgow in 1922, he took part in a seminar with Ballantyne, Eardley Holland and Louise McIlroy on stillbirths and neonatal deaths. In 1921 he was invited to join the Medical Research Council as a part-time researcher and received grants for investigations, in collaboration with Dr WR Logan, into the causes of abortion and intra-uterine death. There followed, in 1923 and 1924, studies of intranatal infection, the biochemical changes in pre-eclampsia and a major project: the estimation of age, weight and length of normal fetuses, and the weight of their organs, in over 600 fetuses delivered at various stages of pregnancy. He had been admitted to the Fellowship of the Edinburgh Obstetrical Society in 1919 and became a regular attender and presenter of papers at the Society's meetings. In due course he was appointed editor of the *Transactions* of the Society.

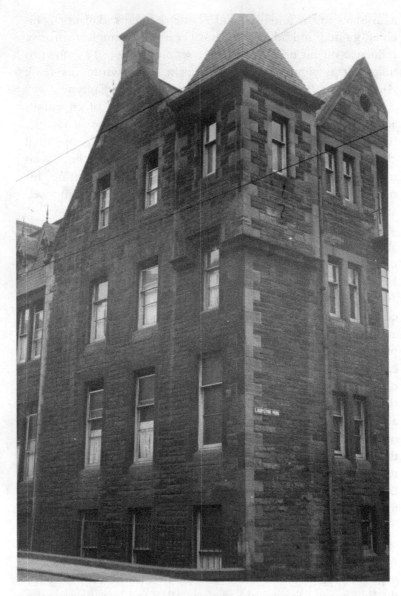

The Royal Edinburgh Maternity and Simpson Memorial Hospital

In 1923 FJ applied for the post of assistant physician to the Edinburgh Royal Infirmary and the Simpson Memorial Pavilion. In his application, he stated:

In 1920 I assisted Dr Ballantyne in the organisation of the new indoor department in the Milne-Murray wing of the Hospital, and have since been associated with him in the care of the patients admitted there for treatment. I have thus been able to acquire a large clinical experience of the abnormalities and diseases of pregnancy... It was impossible for anyone to have been so closely associated with the late Dr Ballantyne, whose fame as the pioneer in prematernity care was world wide, without imbibing some of his enthusiasm, approaching somewhat to his outlook on the present-day problems of the practice and teaching of obstetrics, and benefiting very largely by his unique experience.

With his application he submitted references and testimonials from the most eminent authorities. Ballantyne (who died that year) praised his contributions to obstetrics and gynaecology and referred to his 'sterling quality of frankness, fairness and loyalty. He has an infectious enthusiasm for his work and in his writing he marshals his facts with logical accuracy and force'. Other testimonials came from James Young, RW Johnstone, William Fordyce, Haig Ferguson and others. He was duly appointed.

In that year there were 1,559 deliveries, with 39 maternal deaths (2.3%) and 189 stillbirths and neonatal deaths of whom only 67 were full-term. The high maternal mortality was typical of obstetrics in those days, with sepsis, eclampsia, hyperemesis, placenta praevia and accidental haemorrhage as the main causes. Clinical duties and research now became FJ's main priorities. In addition, he was recognised as the outstanding teacher of medical students in Edinburgh. His wide experience of midwifery in Abertillery gave him special insight into the problems they would face as general practitioners, who at that time presided over most deliveries. At the same time his wide knowledge of obstetrics and gynaecology placed him in high demand as teacher of post-graduates.

In 1925 FJ was awarded the Edinburgh DSc (Doctor of Science) degree and was promoted to Chief Physician, a post he would hold for only a short time.

Notes

1 Letter to Ballantyne 28 November 1918.
2 *Edinburgh Medical Journal* 1920;25:296–307.

Chapter Four

University College Hospital
1926–1946

Francis Browne was appointed Professor at the University of London and Director of the newly established Obstetric Unit of University College Hospital in 1926 and held the post until his retirement in 1946.

The appointment of an Irishman, qualified in Scotland and after 13 years in general practice in Wales to such a post is remarkable. Most appointments to London teaching hospitals at that time would have been of graduates and former residents of the hospital itself. FJ was appointed not by invitation but following his application for the post which was advertised as full-time. Full-time appointments to independent hospitals were rare in those days and it is not known what the field of applicants was. However, his midwifery experience in Abertillery, his previous appointment as Obstetrician to the Edinburgh Royal Infirmary, his research, particularly into miscarriage and stillbirth and his reputation as a teacher would have stood him in good stead. He had also organised the new antenatal department of the Edinburgh Royal Infirmary: no such facility existed at UCH at that time.

It is necessary to discuss briefly the development of medical student training at that time.

The Council of London University was formally appointed in 1826 and land was purchased at the northern end of Gower Street for a college and a hospital. The college was opened in 1828 and medical tuition commenced. A dispensary was opened in 1828, but the real hospital (originally known as the North London, later as University College Hospital) with accommodation for 130 patients was not opened until 1834. David Davis (1777–1841), a graduate from Glasgow, was the first Professor of Midwifery appointed to the College in 1827. He had already achieved fame as the physician–accoucheur who had safely delivered the Duchess of Kent of a daughter in 1819 – the future Queen Victoria. This was only two years after the tragic confinement of Princess Charlotte, daughter of the Prince Regent and second in line of succession to the throne. She was delivered, after a prolonged labour, of a stillborn child and died herself from postpartum haemorrhage the next day. Her obstetrician, Sir Richard Croft, subsequently committed suicide. These events had attracted much attention in the press and in society and so Davis's reputation became firmly established. When appointed to UCH, Davis had only a small number of obstetric beds (probably three) in the main hospital. His published work is mainly concerned with the obstetric forceps and other instruments.[1]

The hospital soon proved inadequate for the numbers of patients and students wishing to attend and a new hospital was opened on the same site in 1905. Financially the college was responsible for the hospital; this burden became too great and separation became essential to enable the college to balance its books. With the help of donations, a separate clinical medical school was opened and in 1907 both hospital and medical school were placed under the control of a new board of governors. Even then, financially, neither the medical school nor the hospital could function adequately without the input of a great deal of capital. This was provided by a generous donation from the Rockefeller Foundation in 1920. The Foundation, instituted in 1913, had for its purpose 'the well being of Mankind'. Two emissaries from the Foundation came to Europe in 1919. Initially they approached Oxford University as a likely recipient of a donation.[2] They became frustrated by long delays in the negotiations because the Oxford colleges insisted on each having their own say and there was no mechanism for a university agreement without collegiate sanction. The adversarial relationship between individual college councils and the central university administration had long been a brake on the rapid reaching of decisions. (This was highlighted as recently as 1963 by the Robbins report.) Oxford's loss was UCH's gain and Oxford had to wait nearly two decades until the munificence of Lord Nuffield established its clinical chairs. The agreement, concluded in December 1920, between the Rockefeller Foundation and the UCH Board of Governors donated £4 million, with a further £435,000 for maintenance, for the expansion of the surgical and medical units, adequate accommodation for clinical and research laboratories, new residents' quarters, a new nurses' home and eventually the building of a new obstetric hospital.[3]

A Royal Commission on university education in London had recommended in 1913 the establishment of clinical professorial units in the London medical schools. (It was this proposal which had attracted the attention of the Rockefeller Foundation.) Each unit was to have a director, two or three assistants, facilities for laboratory work and research, and also undertake formal teaching of medical students. Previously such teaching had been incidental to the life and work of busy consultants. A meeting of the UCH Faculty of Medicine in 1914 recommended that the directors heading the clinical units should be full-time professors with no right to private practice. These recommendations were shelved during the 1914–1918 war when there were too few beds and insufficient space for their implementation. In fact they were not put into practice until after receipt of the Rockefeller bequest. Medical and surgical units were established in 1920, but there were too few beds and too little accommodation for an obstetric unit.

Dr TR Elliott, an outstandingly able clinician and researcher, was appointed in 1920 as first director of the medical unit. He considered that the unit should maintain a balance between teaching, research and the training of future specialists. The manner in which he organised his unit became a model for other clinical units at UCH and in other centres. He retired in 1938 and was succeeded by Dr (later Sir) Harold Himsworth (1905–1993). The surgical unit was also established in 1920 with Professor CC Choyce as first director, to be succeeded from 1935 to 1937 by the renowned surgeon–philosopher Wilfred Trotter.

The foundation stone of the new Obstetric Hospital in Huntley Street was laid by King George V in 1923. Until this time the provision of obstetric services was entirely geared towards home deliveries. The Board of Governors planned a new start for obstetric care and student teaching. Neither of the two obstetric physicians, George Blacker and Herbert Spencer, wished to undertake the role of director of the new unit. Herbert Spencer MD, FRCP (1887–1925) was emeritus professor at the medical school, but was about to retire and certainly did not want a full-time appointment. So the post was advertised in 1925; FJ Browne was appointed and came to London as the first full-time director of the new obstetric unit. His annual salary was £2,000 a year plus superannuation. Whilst reasonably adequate in 1926, there was no increase during FJ's tenure, despite the pressures of inflation and rising cost of living.

The Obstetric Hospital was at last opened by the Prince of Wales in 1926. FJ started work there on 1 July that year. He brought with him, from Edinburgh, Gladys Dodds (1898–1982), his research assistant, and, four months later, Miss Watson who had been the senior midwifery sister at the Simpson. Chassar Moir (1900–1977) was soon to follow. FJ had no say in the planning of the new Obstetric Hospital. The architects had had little knowledge or experience of the needs of a modern obstetric unit. When completed, it contained antenatal, lying-in and gynaecological beds, labour wards and its own operating theatre, as well as limited laboratory accommodation and teaching facilities. However, there were no antenatal or child welfare clinics, inadequate bedpan sterilising facilities, and no accommodation for medical students or residents: they used to climb over the roof of the residents' building to get to the labour ward for attending

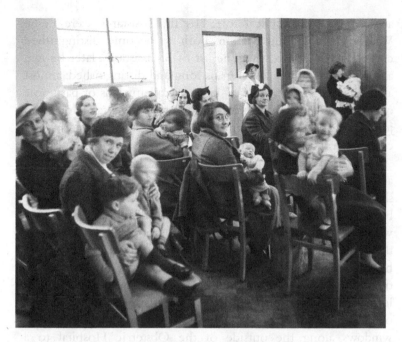
A baby clinic in the obstetric unit at
University College Hospital, c.1928

emergencies at night. Nurseries were inadequate. Initially the
labour wards were disorganised because there was one on each
floor, intended to serve the lying-in beds and supervised by the
sister of that floor. A unified labour ward policy and management
protocols were thus impossible to achieve. FJ had the vision and
drive to overcome these handicaps. Eventually a properly
organised delivery suite was organised on the fourth floor, to
allow for supervision by one senior sister and the introduction of
modern labour ward techniques, including the elimination of
sepsis and the provision of adequate anaesthesia.

FJ's first tasks were to organise the teaching of medical
students, institute antenatal and postnatal clinics, and train assistants who were expected to undertake teaching and research in

addition to their clinical role. His first assistants were Leslie Williams and Harold Malkin, both to become distinguished consultants in due course. The list of his assistants, later known as lecturers or senior lecturers, is long and distinguished: almost all of them later became well-known academicians or part-time consultants. Among the most famous were Chassar Moir who joined the obstetric unit in 1929 and Max Rosenheim who came from the medical unit to the obstetric unit in 1934.

Chassar Moir, whom FJ knew from the Edinburgh days, was among the greatest members of his profession. Tall, slim, with sharp features, long fingers and beautiful hands, he was one of the best teachers and examiners, and a most distinguished speaker with perfect choice of words and an amazing ability to delineate the character and features of his seniors. During his time at UCH he developed techniques to measure intra-uterine pressure and the strength of uterine contractions. For this, small balloons were introduced into the uterine cavity and, in a manner reminiscent of Heath Robinson, were connected by wires passed through windows along the outside of the Obstetric Hospital to a recording manometer in a remote and minute research room. The manometer recorded the tracings of the contractions on a slowly rotating drum.

Once the technique was established, he went on to his great work on ergometrine. Ergotamine and ergotoxine were previously considered the active constituents of liquid extract of ergot. Moir showed that more powerful contractions with more rapid onset resulted from administering the tincture than from the combined effects of the two known alkaloids alone.

From the tincture a hitherto unknown substance was isolated by him and Dr HW Dudley and later purified by Sir Henry Dale at the National Institute of Medical Research. It was called ergo-metrine. It has ever since played a crucial role in the prevention and treatment of postpartum haemorrhage, previously one of the most important causes of maternal death. Moir left the obstetric unit in 1935 to become Reader, later Nuffield Professor, in Oxford. A great obstetrician and gynaecological surgeon, he made major contributions by his work on X-ray pelvimetry (measuring the size of the bony pelvis at various levels which have to be traversed by the fetus during labour) and the management of vesico-vaginal fistula, the cause of that most distressing condition, total urinary incontinence.

Max Rosenheim was seconded from the medical unit in 1934. He introduced mandelic acid for the treatment of urinary tract infections. Previously such infections and especially pyelonephritis had been important causes of maternal morbidity and mortality; termination of pregnancy had to be performed in some intractable cases to preserve the pregnant woman's life. It was already known that a ketogenic diet used for epilepsy led to the appearance in the urine of keto-acids and an environment in which the bacteria responsible for urinary tract infections could not survive. Mandelic acid became widely and successfully used until the introduction of sulphonamides and later antibiotics. Rosenheim had a distinguished army career during the war and later became Director of the Medical Unit and Professor of Medicine after the resignation of Sir Harold Himsworth. He became a Fellow of the Royal Society, President of the Royal College of Physicians and a peer.

Other assistants included Norman White and Tim Flew who both became consultants at UCH, Robert (later Professor) Kellar, Vivian Barnett, Fouracre Barnes, Aileen Dickens and Josephine (later Dame Josephine) Barnes. Throughout this time, Gladys Dodds worked in the obstetric unit and was an indefatigable researcher. Her publications on urinary tract infections in pregnancy and the numerous investigations into pregnancy toxaemias and their ultimate prognosis which she undertook with FJ are outstanding.

The atmosphere at UCH in those days was electric. Sir Thomas Lewis, consultant physician and member of the Medical Research Council, had been the first to develop the concepts of clinical science and research on patients. Previously research had centred mainly on anatomy, physiology and pathology. Lewis, Professor TR Elliott and Professor Wilfred Trotter – all three

Fellows of the Royal Society – were FJ's contemporaries. He would meet them almost daily at lunch in the refectory where consultants and professors were seated at the 'top table' and had an opportunity of exchanging views. Browne was well aware of the rapid advances in medicine and especially in the art and science of surgery since the introduction by Lister of measures to prevent and control infection. There had been no corresponding improvements in the practice of obstetrics. Puerperal sepsis (childbed fever) remained the major cause of maternal mortality. FJ set himself the task of improving the practice of obstetrics by better training of students and midwives, the introduction of aseptic techniques in the delivery suite and the strict separation of 'dirty' from 'clean' cases.

The new Obstetric Hospital had ten antenatal and 30 lying-in beds, as well as 30 gynaecological beds. Soon after its opening, deliveries in hospital reached the number of about 800 per year with more than 200 antenatal admissions. The number of deliveries increased to about 1000 a year until the war started in 1939. After the war and in FJ's last year before retirement in 1946 there were 1178 deliveries. This was at the time the largest number of deliveries undertaken in any of the London teaching hospitals. It has to be remembered that in those days women were nursed for seven to ten days in the lying-in wards and so the number of deliveries in relation to the number of beds is totally different from present practice. FJ reached an agreement with the part-time consultants that the staff of the obstetric unit should be responsible for all obstetrics and that the gynaecological work should be shared.

One of Professor Browne's duties was to submit Annual Reports to the Dean of the Medical School. Copies of these have been preserved and I was kindly given access to them by Professor Charles Rodeck. Starting in 1926, they record the institution of four antenatal clinics a week instead of one, and of weekly postnatal clinics. The labour wards were for the first time put under the charge of one senior sister and new techniques were introduced. These included quite elementary practices like wearing masks, scrubbing hands and wearing surgical gloves, gowns and clean boots. Systematic teaching of medical students was started, consisting of 60 lectures in one 12-week term, ward rounds and bedside teaching. Students spent two months as obstetric 'dressers', one on the district, followed by attendance as gynaecological dresser. They attended antenatal clinics and gynaecological operations. Browne insisted on accurate record keeping. He considered this, with accurate description of findings on vaginal examinations, obstetric procedures and gynaecological operations, to be the essence of good teaching. The wide range of these changes show that FJ knew exactly what he wanted to achieve, and that hard work and long hours did not deter him.

In 1927, ten additional lying-in beds were opened; arrangements were made for students to live in and a study room was provided for them on the top floor of the Obstetric Hospital. Research projects included work by FJ and Gladys Dodds on accidental haemorrhage, and FJ with Joan Taylor on the bacteriology of puerperal sepsis. The 1928 report records the visit of Dr Bruce Mayes from Sydney and FJ's visit to ten centres in the USA and Canada at the invitation of the Rockefeller Foundation. Such tours and visits to overseas institutions were a major undertaking in those days before the advent of relatively cheap commercial air flights. Arrangements were made for fully trained midwives instead of 'handy women' to accompany students on the district. This resulted in halving the number of cases of puerperal infection. In 1929, Chassar Moir became Unit Assistant. A ten-bedded observation ward for patients suspected of infection was opened. Equipment for the provision of general anaesthesia was obtained for the labour wards. In 1930 new protocols were introduced for nurses and midwives in the labour wards. In 1931 there is reference to the research with Gladys Dodds on pregnancy toxaemia and the outcome of pregnancy in women who developed urinary tract infections or toxaemia in pregnancy. Following Norman White's appointment as consultant, Chassar Moir became first assistant in 1932 and his work on uterine contractions and the isolation of ergometrine occupy much of the 1934/35 reports. Rosenheim's introduction of mandelic acid is detailed as is also the first publication of FJ's book *Antenatal and Postnatal Care*.

In 1936, Sister Watson, who had accompanied FJ from Edinburgh, retired. Monthly regular staff meetings were introduced, paving the way to the present-day audits. In 1937, JDS Flew was first assistant and JGH Ince joined the unit and started his studies of different pelvic types. In 1938, Gladys Dodds became first assistant. Arrangements were completed for some of the medical students to spend time and do deliveries at St Mary's Hospital, Islington. In 1939, FJ completed the third edition of *Antenatal and Postnatal Care* and started work on the detection in early pregnancy of patients predisposed to later development of toxaemia. 1940 saw, due to the war, the posting of students to various hospitals in the district and the Obstetric Hospital was briefly evacuated. Later, hospital deliveries were resumed with a much reduced number of 653; they took place in the basement because of the threat of bombs. The 1941 report speaks of the taking over of the hospital by the Emergency Medical Services to provide for the possible treatment of wounded. Teaching was difficult as the antenatal beds were moved to Hemel Hempstead and Watford and many of the assistants were away on war service. 1942 saw the arrival of Josephine Barnes from Chassar Moir's unit at Oxford and she soon became first assistant when Fouracre Barnes joined the armed forces. With a depleted staff it was a hard struggle to maintain standards of teaching and clinical management. FJ held a clinic once a week at the Watford Peace Memorial Hospital. His rounds there were attended by large numbers of students. The four lower floors of the Obstetric Hospital were reopened, but it was still difficult to provide enough deliveries for the students and they were sent out to Hackney and Nottingham. FJ brought out the 4th edition of *Antenatal and Postnatal Care* and he and Gladys Dodds published an important study of pregnancy in patients with chronic hypertension. In 1943 full teaching was resumed at the Obstetric Hospital. Aileen Dickens was appointed assistant. Obstetric and gynaecological training of students was reduced from six to three months in the students' curriculum. FJ saw this as a most unfavourable move but it was made necessary by the expanding range of the teaching syllabus and acknowledged the trend that the majority of deliveries in the country now took place in hospital, so that knowledge of obstetrics was no longer such a significant requirement for general practitioners. The year 1944 saw the opening of the Western Front in Europe and the menace of flying bombs. Teaching continued with difficulty under these circumstances. FJ published the fifth edition of *Antenatal and Postnatal Care* and started his work with Josephine Barnes on hypertension in pregnancy. One part of their research was to take the blood pressure of patients' mothers and sisters whilst they were visiting patients in hospital, to determine whether there was a hereditary element in gestational hypertension.

In the 1945 report, FJ again stresses the problems of a depleted staff which made adequate teaching and research difficult. He himself carried much of the teaching burden and the year also saw the 6th edition of his book and the beginning of his work on pressor substances.

FJ's last report was written in 1946. In this, he states that staffing levels had returned to normal and teaching had become more satisfactory. Josephine Barnes's study on the use of pethidine in labour is mentioned with pride. FJ had long worked to improve methods of analgesia and anaesthesia in labour. He used this – the last report before his retirement – to summarise what he thought were his main achievements in his 20 years as director of the obstetric unit:

- the modernisation of labour ward techniques and equipment, of the lying-in and antenatal wards and of the district work
- the introduction, in 1938, of an obstetric flying squad to attend emergencies over a large area of north London
- the reorganisation of medical student teaching

- the systematic training of pupil midwives
- the training of future specialists
- research which culminated in 80 papers and 18 books (including new editions) by his assistants and himself; Chassar Moir's work on ergometrine and Gladys Dodds's on urinary tract infections are specifically mentioned
- the institution of a 'toxaemia clinic' with improved and more conscientious standards of antenatal care.

Notes

1 Davis DD. *The Principles and Practice of Obstetric Medicine in a Series of Systematic Dissertations on the Diseases of Women and Children, Volumes 1–3*. London: Taylor and Walton; 1836.
2 Annan, N. *The Dons*. London: Harper Collins; 1999.
3 Merrington, MR. *University College Hospital and the Medical School*. London: William Heinemann; 1976.

Chapter Five

FJ Browne –
teacher, clinician and researcher

FJ's ability as a teacher was renowned. In his first academic appointment in Edinburgh his reputation spread quickly, and indeed provided a necessary addition to a low income. This reputation was one of the qualities which led to his appointment at UCH where teaching undergraduates was his primary task. Following his retirement, he devoted more of his time to teaching postgraduates in London. It was the high regard he had earned as a teacher which gained him consultant appointments at three hospitals in Sydney when he settled to live in Australia.

Three major influences led to this excellence. His practice in Abertillery as a general practitioner and miners' doctor taught him the need to learn and practise obstetric skills, which were in particular need when most deliveries were done by general practitioners in patients' own homes. In his work at Edinburgh, he was enormously influenced by John Ballantyne whose vision was that obstetric mishaps and tragedies could be prevented by antenatal care. Finally his own personality and upbringing was an important factor. Parental examples of hard work, intellectual honesty, a serious approach to life and sharing in the life of the local community, together with the ethos of excellent schooling and religious faith, combined to produce a man of intelligence and integrity with a deep sense of responsibility. It is worth noting that all his siblings did well in their chosen careers: two of his sisters became nurses, and one, Matilda, became a hospital matron. The schools to which his

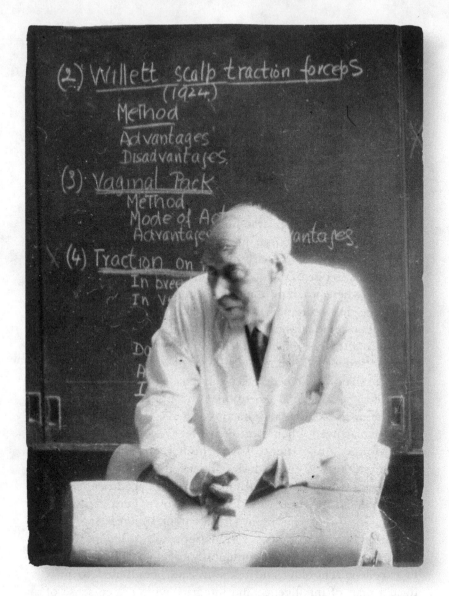

FJ Browne lecturing at University College Hospital, c. 1938
(by an unknown student)

parents sent him were chosen as the best available and were known for the calibre of the teachers. In addition, there is no doubt that a well-developed religious background helped to instil the necessary characteristics and standards which were maintained in later life. The family were Presbyterians and the strict discipline and seriousness of this religion were impressed on the young man and became permanent features of his outlook and way of life.

Teaching in clinical medicine has many different aspects. Teaching obstetric students is bound to be didactic, embracing both the theory and the practice of obstetrics. Teaching in FJ's time was entirely by ward rounds and lectures. At this level, there is little opportunity for a one-to-one relationship between teacher and pupil and the quality of the teaching depends entirely on the personality and skills of the teacher. The first necessity is to have an expert and intimate knowledge of the subject. The second is to be able to capture the interest and stimulate the imagination of the audience. FJ had these abilities and was an excellent communicator, as is indicated by his body language and posture whilst lecturing. In his case nothing could have been further from the truth than the old adage that 'lectures are a means of transferring information from the notebook of the lecturer to that of the student without passing through the brain of either'. Finally, the good teacher instils good habits and sets an example which persists throughout a doctor's life.

Teaching a resident who is concerned with the day-to-day care of patients is entirely different. It affords an opportunity to teach the finer details of diagnosis, management and prognosis as well as ways of communication, in which the art of listening is as important as responding. This requires more of a one-to-one relationship and is of greatest importance to the development of a doctor.

Senior assistants or lecturers again require a different approach: they need to be guided to use their clinical skills, be taught scientific methods and the use of libraries and allowed to develop and pursue their own interests.

For the medical students and residents, FJ's greatest achievement was the publication in 1935 of the first edition of *Antenatal and Postnatal Care*. This book was the first of its kind: previous obstetric texts had concentrated on labour and delivery, but there were no earlier books on the care of women in pregnancy. At the time it was first written, most deliveries were at the patient's home, supervised by midwives and general practitioners. The purpose of the book was to provide training and instructions for them. From conception until delivery, all physiological changes and abnormalities or diseases encountered in pregnant women are described and their management is discussed. The text is comprehensive, clearly written and easy to assimilate. The style is crisp, succinct and precise with short clear sentences – a tribute to good schooling with its teaching of grammar and self-expression. It smacks of an era when EBM stood for expressed breast milk rather than evidence based medicine, and issues became clear even before the invention of meta-analysis. The impact of this book was instant and enormous. It became essential reading for many generations of medical students and residents. Although techniques of diagnosis and management have inevitably changed greatly since then, the text still makes enjoyable reading and provides a good source of information about the evolution of these changes. The dedication reads:

'To the Memory of my late chief and friend John William Ballantyne, pioneer in Antenatal Pathology and Antenatal Care in grateful remembrance of many kindnesses.'

There is no doubt that Ballantyne was the great visionary who believed that better antenatal care would reduce the incidence of maternal and fetal mortality and morbidity. His influence on FJ's development was enormous. FJ had the same vision and the ability and determination to apply the principles propounded by Ballantyne in practice. FJ's main interest always was in obstetrics and his main passion was the teaching of it to his medical students. He believed that the obstetric side of training was by far the more important for general practitioners and that gynaecology could safely be left to the specialist. He himself did relatively little gynaecological work or operations. This was largely the domain of his senior assistants and the part-time consultants during his time at UCH. Practice has changed greatly since those days: now the great majority of deliveries take place in hospital under the supervision of residents and consultants. On the other hand, training the general practitioner in medical gynaecology has become ever more important for the management of hormonal problems, infertility, contraception, infections and many general gynaecological complaints.

In 1946, FJ reached the age of compulsory retirement from the Chair at UCH. This is a difficult period in anybody's life and the change from full activity to a life of inactivity can be one of the hardest adjustments to be made. Henry, his younger son, had been killed during the war and the other three children had left home. The greatest blow was Minnie's prolonged illness, leading to her death in 1948 from malignant disease. The combined effect of retirement and the loss of his life's partner were shattering blows. FJ responded, as he always had, by immersing himself in work. He joined the staff of the Watford Peace Memorial Hospital, not far from his home, and advised on obstetrics in general and antenatal care specifically. He also started teaching classes for postgraduates aspiring to pass the MRCOG (Membership of the Royal College of Obstetricians and Gynaecologists) examination. The classes were held at the Soho Hospital for Women and the City of London Maternity Hospital. Mr Elliot Philipp attended such a class and says the teaching was excellent and contained material not published elsewhere. There would be about 20 students per class, many of them from abroad. The teaching was fluent and not didactic; lectures were delivered clearly at speeds which the non-English students could follow and make adequate notes. Complex issues were explained in a simple manner. 'All in all, he was considered a wonderful teacher.'

These postgraduate lectures became the basis of his book *Postgraduate Obstetrics and Gynaecology*. The first edition was published in 1950 with FJ as sole author. In the Preface he says 'the aim of a teacher should be, I think, to know the literature so far as he can, to filter it through his mind and give his conclusions, right or wrong. An article or a book read, a chat at tea time with a friend, a bitter experience that has burnt into the mind – it is these that make up the sum total of anyone's experience and of that which is embodied in this book'. The second edition, published in 1955, was published jointly with his son, John McClure Browne, who by this time had become Professor of Obstetrics and Gynaecology at the Institute of Obstetrics and Gynaecology, and Head of Department at the Postgraduate Medical School of London. It bears evidence of FJ's new domicile in Australia and some of the great obstetricians and gynaecologists he had got to know there. For many generations of MRCOG candidates and aspiring specialists, this book became essential and highly rewarding reading.

Medical students crowded into his lectures and provided large and attentive audiences at his weekly ward rounds. Many of his writings, directed mainly at them, filled the pages of the *University College Hospital Magazine*, in which he attempted to explain principles of training. Much active teaching of obstetrics takes place in the middle of the night by specialists called in to attend an emergency which may present the ideal opportunity to teach students as well as provide expert assistance to the patient and her baby. FJ insisted that such labour ward teaching was an essential part of student training.

A glance at the bibliography at the end of this volume reveals something of FJ's research interests. These range from individual case reports to wider subjects which required active research. His work on accidental haemorrhage (believed to be associated with chronic nephritis) led to experimental work on rabbits. His detailed studies, mainly undertaken in his Edinburgh days, on stillbirth and neonatal death and on postmaturity and syphilis in pregnancy did much to establish his reputation early in his career. However, throughout his life, his main interest, for which his research was chiefly remembered, was in pre-eclampsia and much of his time was spent on improving antenatal care for the early diagnosis of pregnancy hypertension and pre-eclampsia. Again and again he came back to discuss theories of aetiology and prognosis, which remain highly controversial even today. He himself came to the conclusion that excessive pituitary and adrenal cortical function, together with placental ischaemia, were the main aetiological factors. As far as future prognosis is concerned, he was greatly assisted in his long-term follow-up studies of affected patients by Gladys Dodds and later Josephine Barnes. The old view, that 30% of patients with pre-eclampsia developed chronic nephritis, was proved wrong. Women who developed chronic hypertension after an eclamptic pregnancy, he concluded, would have become hypertensive anyway and pregnancy acted as precursor rather than cause. It is of little surprise that when he was chosen to deliver the highly prestigious William Fletcher Shaw Memorial Oration at the Royal College of Obstetricians and Gynaecologists in 1947, he chose hypertension in pregnancy as his subject. He returned to this theme in one of his last papers, read to a meeting on hypertension and pregnancy toxaemias, in Sydney in 1957.

On a slightly different plane, a large part of his teaching took the form of lectures and seminars, aimed at both professionals and administrators. The more eminent he became, the more he was in demand to speak on broader issues such as the teaching of obstetrics, the organisation of obstetric services in the country and the part played by education of medical students.

Among other clinical interests, FJ set up the first flying squad service in London, following the example of Frank Stabler in Newcastle. Fully equipped teams consisting of a midwife, an obstetrician, a house surgeon and a medical student were always on standby to assist with any emergencies encountered in domiciliary practice. Postpartum haemorrhage, undiagnosed breech presentation, unexpected twin delivery, maternal and fetal distress were the main indications for calling out the flying squad. Most emergency treatment, including cross-matching blood and transfusion, was administered in the patient's home and only a few cases were transferred to hospital. During his time as Director of the UCH Obstetric Unit, Chassar Moir, then his assistant, did his great work on the isolation of ergometrine which led not only to improved treatment for postpartum haemorrhage but later became almost universally used for the prevention of this life threatening condition. Also under his directorship, his assistant Josephine Barnes did her important work on pethidine.

Relief of pain before, during and after delivery was then, as it still is, one of the most important aspects of obstetric practice. Pain associated with uterine contractions in labour was first seriously relieved by James Young Simpson (1811–1870), who introduced chloroform and ether to replace older more homely remedies, and administered the former to Queen Victoria in 1853 for her eighth delivery. However these drugs were usually used only during the second stage of labour and morphine, scopolamine and later nitrous oxide and air and trilene remained the standard drugs used in the first stage. It was in the 1930s that Grantly Dick-Read first attempted to make childbirth once more a natural process which did not require pain relieving drugs. He was an obstetrician who worked mainly in private practice in the 1930–1950 era and was well known as a prolific writer and lecturer. His many books included *Natural Childbirth*, *The Revelation of Childbirth* and *Childbirth without Fear* and were the precursors of a whole new movement in obstetrics. They were based on the theory that apprehension and the fear of pain were the cause of failure to relax and of abnormal muscle tension ('tense mind – tense cervix') and that they could be overcome by antenatal teaching of the physiology of labour and techniques of relaxation.

FJ invited Dick-Read to write the chapters 'Pain in childbirth' and 'The influence of the emotions upon pregnancy and parturition' in the earlier editions of *Antenatal and Postnatal Care*. But it is noteworthy that FJ changed his outlook and embraced newer approaches as they came along. Dick-Read's chapters became shorter and shorter in later editions. While preparing the second edition of *Postgraduate Obstetrics and Gynaecology*, letters were exchanged between FJ (then in Australia) and John McClure Browne on the subject.[1] Dick-Read by then was only briefly mentioned with more space given to descriptions of the use of pethidine, and caudal and epidural anaesthesia. Perhaps the last word on the subject remains with Chassar Moir, who described the agony of a patient with cervical dystocia: distressed and uncontrollable, 'she was given an epidural anaesthetic and so relaxed and took from her locker her copy of *Natural Childbirth* and contentedly read another chapter'. It was during FJ's time as Director of the UCH Obstetric Unit that Josephine Barnes first introduced pethidine which became the standard obstetric analgesic for the next fifty years. FJ also introduced the use of local anaesthetics for the performance of episiotomy and for vaginal repair after delivery. Painful stitches have always been a cause of much maternal discomfort, especially for mothers sitting to breastfeed their babies.

Note

1   Letter from John to FJ, 18 September 1953.

Chapter Six

A Member and A Fellow

FJ was both a member of the Gynaecological Visiting Society and a Fellow[1] of the Royal Society of Medicine. Election to membership of the former and attainment of office in the latter are singular distinctions as they indicate recognition by one's fellows and peers, outweighing recognition by other, sometimes more elevated, bodies.

The Gynaecological Visiting Society (GVS) is the oldest and perhaps most prestigious of the 'gynaecological clubs'. It was founded in 1911 by Professor William Blair-Bell of Liverpool and some of his colleagues as a visiting society in order to provide for members 'the encouragement and demonstration of scientific research and the study of methods employed in gynaecological clinics'. Ordinary membership was restricted to 30 with preference given to those engaged in research. Those elected were mainly young, energetic and leading members of the profession. Two centres were to be visited each year, one of them preferably abroad. The Society soon became renowned because of the distinguished membership which included, among others, Blair-Bell, Munro Kerr, Comyns Berkeley, Victor Bonney, Eardley Holland and Aleck Bourne, as well as for the high standards of the clinical programmes and the excellence of the dinners. The original subscription was £1 a year.

It is of particular interest to note that two members of the GVS, William Fletcher Shaw and Blair-Bell, first conceived the idea of a College of Obstetricians and Gynaecologists, similar to the Royal Colleges of Physician and Surgeons. The GVS was in many ways the parent of the College when it was finally opened

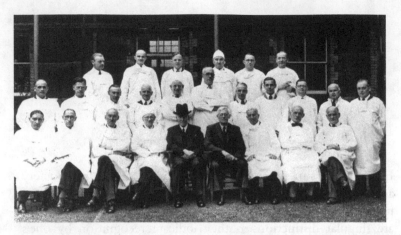

The Cardiff meeting of the Gynaecological Visiting Society in
September 1948. FJ is seated third from the left in the front row

in 1929 as the College of Obstetricians and Gynaecologists,
receiving its Royal Charter in 1937. It would be a fair assessment
of the GVS's contribution that the Society played a crucial role
in bringing about the transition from the art of midwifery to the
science of obstetrics.

FJ was elected to GVS membership at Sheffield in 1927 and
attended his first meeting as a new member in Belfast in 1928
where he was introduced to the rites of the Society and experienced his first tasting of vintage wines.

The London members entertained the Society in 1929 and
the programme included talks by FJ on accidental haemorrhage
at the Obstetric Hospital and surgical demonstrations at the
Samaritan Hospital by Clifford White, William Gilliatt, Aleck
Bourne (who did a total hysterectomy with removal of the
appendages in under 30 minutes) and Victor Bonney who did
his 381st Wertheim operation in 50 minutes.

FJ attended meetings in Bristol (1930) where the programme
included a visit to Harveys' cellars, Liverpool (1931) when a
financial crisis dominated the meeting and other meetings in the

UK as well as in Germany, Switzerland, Holland, Vienna and Budapest. However, his membership lapsed in 1935 when he had failed to attend three consecutive meetings. He was reinstated as an Honorary Member – a unique distinction – at the first post-war meeting in Oxford in 1945.

Following his death in 1963, an outstanding and most moving tribute was paid to JF by Chassar Moir at the 107th meeting of the GVS.

FJ became a Foundation Fellow of the College of Obstetricians and Gynaecologists when it was first established in 1929 and continued as an active member all his life. He was co-opted on to Council as a Fellows' Representative for London from 1945 to 1947 and also was a member of the Maternal and Infant

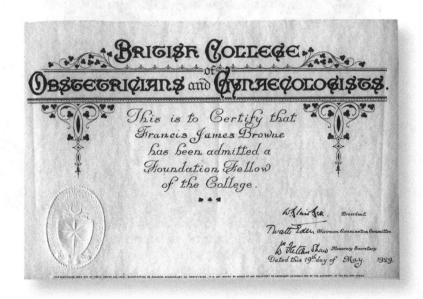

The Foundation Fellow's certificate presented to FJ Browne
on 19 May 1929

Health Services Committee from 1945 to 1947 and of the Joint Committee with the British Paediatric Neonatal Committee from 1945 to 1946. These were important times in the development of British obstetric services, leading to the introduction of the National Health Service, the tendency towards hospital in preference to domiciliary deliveries, and the establishment of the highest standards of teaching, examining and appointment of would-be specialists.

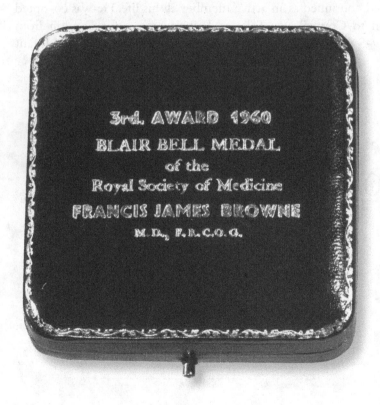

The dedication on the presentation case for the Blair-Bell medal, awarded to FJ Browne in 1960

In 1947, FJ was awarded the first William Meredith Fletcher Shaw Memorial lectureship, a distinction bestowed by the College on a highly esteemed members of the profession. FJ's chosen title was 'Hypertension in pregnancy' and he recorded a lifetime's research.

FJ joined the Royal Society of Medicine (RSM) when he came to London and soon was elected a member of the Section of Obstetrics and Gynaecology.

The origins of the RSM go back to the foundation of the Medical Society of London in 1773. This was incorporated into the Medical and Chirurgical Society of London in 1805 and awarded the Royal Charter in 1834, despite fierce opposition from the Royal College of Physicians. In 1907 the Royal Medical and Chirurgical Society joined forces with 15 other – mainly specialised – societies, including the Obstetrical Society of London to become the RSM. The Society moved into purpose built premises at the corner of Wimpole Street and Henrietta Street in 1907, where there are lecture theatres, meeting rooms and dining facilities, but above all housing the Library, one of the finest medical libraries in the world.

The Section of Obstetrics and Gynaecology, continuing the traditions of the Obstetrical Society of London, campaigned for the compulsory education and examination of midwives, culminating in the Midwives Act of 1902 and the ordering of teaching students of obstetrics and gynaecology. It also led the way in the investigation of maternal and infant mortality (subjects close to FJ's heart), eclampsia and puerperal sepsis. The influence of the Section's work was great; in the days before postgraduate education, scientific courses and congresses became everyday events.

FJ was President of the Section of Obstetrics and Gynaecology for the 1945/46 session. His Council reads like a roll of honour. Vice Presidents were Aleck Bourne, Alan Brews, Munro Kerr, Charles Read and Leslie Williams. Other members of council included Douglas MacLeod, Ralph Winterton, Joe Wrigley, Sir Comyns Berkeley, Victor Lack, Percy Malpas,

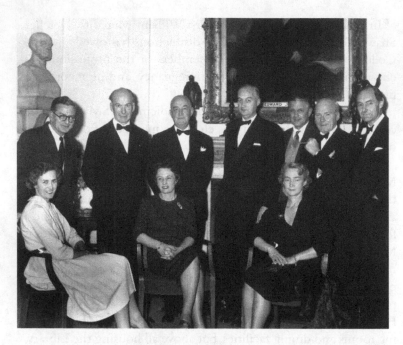

FJ Browne's family at the Blair-Bell presentation ceremony;
Eileen and Robert Mitchell, Veronica and John McClure Browne,
Olive and John Hurford, with Robert Percival and Ralph Winterton

Chassar Moir, John Stallworthy, Gladys Dodds, Josephine Barnes
and Carnac Rivett.

Speakers at meetings in this session included Malcolm Donald-
son on carcinoma of the cervix, Ivor Hughes on rubella in pregnancy, Macafee on placenta praevia, Wrigley on postmaturity and
Nixon and Theobald on water metabolism in pregnancy.

Among those presenting Cases were Stanley Clayton, Hum-
phrey Arthure, William Hawksworth and Braithwaite Rickford.
Much thought and time had gone into assembling such a splendid programme.

FJ's presidential address in October 1945 was not published in
the *Proceedings* of the RSM, but a copy remains in the Australian

archives. It was entitled: 'The obstetric unit: ideals and realities'. In it he describes how the Report of the Royal Commission (the Haldane Commission) led to the establishment of professorial units to improve, and introduce scientific and university standards to, the teaching of medical students. This had to be done by paid teachers who combined clinical care with teaching and active research. Professors were to be appointed in medicine, surgery, and obstetrics and gynaecology who had control of wards and outpatient departments, could appoint assistants and had laboratory accommodation. Teaching and research were to be considered as twin brothers and should stimulate students to think for themselves.

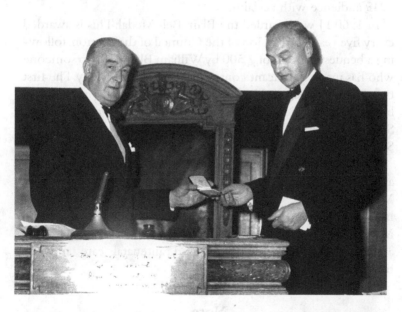

Professor John McClure Browne (right) accepting the Blair-Bell medal on behalf of his father, who was not well enough to make the long journey from Australia, from Harold Malkin (left), in London, 28 October 1960

Having outlined these ideals, FJ then considered how their three-fold purpose of teaching students, training specialists and advancing knowledge could be achieved. Much thought is given to student teaching, to make it interesting, stimulating and 'alive'. Similarly the appointment and training of assistants is discussed in detail. FJ considers whether professors should be allowed private practice (this was not then allowed in the University of London): he considers this necessary to preserve their own clinical experience and pass it on to the students. Finally FJ discusses research and the need to appoint experienced staff such as endocrinologists and biochemists, to solve problems for which their expertise is essential.

Most of these principles are in common practice today, but their need, emphasised so eloquently by FJ, was accepted by his 1945 audience with acclaim.

In 1960 FJ was awarded the Blair-Bell Medal. This is awarded every five years by decision of the Council of the Section, following a bequest in 1936 of £500 by William Blair-Bell, to someone who has made significant contributions to the specialty. The first two recipients before FJ were Munro Kerr and Leonard Colebrook. Later recipients were Charles Macafee, Ian Donald, Patrick Steptoe, Geoffrey Dawes, Alec Turnbull, Kenneth Bagshawe and Sir John Dewhurst.

FJ was too frail to make the journey from Australia and the award was accepted on his behalf by his son, Professor John McClure Browne. FJ's daughters, Olive and Eileen, and their husbands were present. The presentation was made by Harold Malkin who recalled that he was registrar at UCH when FJ arrived in 1926 and revolutionised antenatal care and the training of medical students.

` Note

1   Fellowship was awarded following personal nomination and ballot and signified no specific academic status.

Chapter Seven

The man

FJ was born, bred and remained a Presbyterian. He attended a church where a really good sermon was appreciated. Like his father before him, he was an unusually tall man, being six foot three or four inches in height. He was of sparse build, the result perhaps of a rather frugal diet. His original Aberdeen fare of porridge was followed by lunches of rice pudding consumed at the BMA or the RSM to where, when in London, he walked regularly at lunchtime to catch up with reading. He had twinkling eyes and walked with a slight stoop. His forehead was high, his nose prominent and his slightly bulging eyes seems always to express surprise. In his later years he had a small grey-white moustache and white hair which curled a little upwards in the nape of his neck.

Gentle and kind are the terms repeatedly used to describe FJ by those who knew him. He radiated friendship and had time for other people and the ability to communicate with them, being an animated conversationalist. These are often characteristics of children born into large families and FJ remained a member of his large family all his life. Subsequent generations recall the great distances he would travel to see relations, his sense of humour, how good he was with children, his great personality – and a fondness for cigars after lunch.

He was also highly approachable to his colleagues and junior staff. Peter Fell, his last houseman, specifically recalls that he was always available to any member of his team whether they came

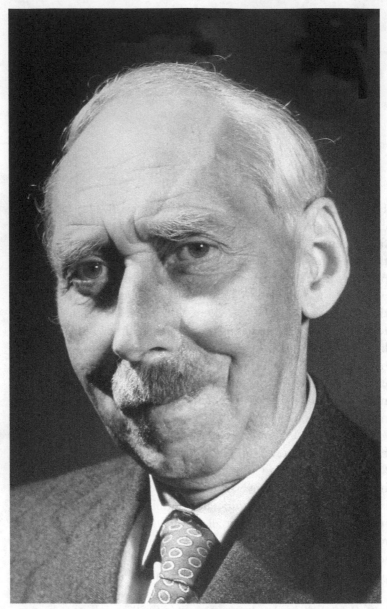

Professor FJ Browne

to him for advice or support. The former requires extensive knowledge and wisdom which could be shared with junior staff; the latter is essential in a demanding and stressful profession and was a further illustration of his kindness. In his days at UCH the professor's office was a small room on the ground floor next to the main entrance – just big enough to house a desk, two chairs and a bookcase. The atmosphere was relatively casual and unofficial. In his successor's day the offices of the Director of the Unit were moved to allow for more space and better facilities – but in the process a certain intimacy was lost.

As John Peel has written, 'F.J. was revered by all his residents, lecturers, registrars and students, not only because of his erudition and teaching, but because he was such a kindly and generous-hearted man.'[1] He was widely acknowledged to be an outstanding teacher and his rapport with undergraduates is indicated by the occasion when he arrived to lecture to find the long desk in the lecture theatre looking like a harvest festival – with millet seeds, grapes, tangerines, walnuts, melons and other fruits. Not batting an eyelid, he thanked the students for their help in illustrating the lecture, likened the fruits to the sizes of various ovarian tumours, ate several of them, remarked that the grapes were particularly sweet and requested that the remaining ones be packed for him to take home!

He was a passionate walker, a habit no doubt dating from his isolated childhood on the farm in Northern Ireland, miles from any form of transport. Five to ten miles meant nothing to him and fifteen-mile walks, and a cold bath in the morning, were standard. In Edinburgh he lived within walking distance of his hospital and place of work. Commuting from Watford to London, when he was professor at UCH, meant a long walk to the station, taking the train from there to Marylebone, and proceeding to the hospital. At lunchtime he could often be seen going without lunch to walk to the libraries at the BMA or, in the opposite direction, the RSM.

FJ had an enormous ability to concentrate and paid great attention to details. He was a prodigious reader and necessarily spent much time keeping up with advances and research in obstetrics and gynaecology, an activity which made him an invaluable reviewer of articles submitted to a wide range of journals. His reading extended well beyond his professional interests. A volume of Gibbon, Walter Scott, Jane Austen or other distinguished classical author was nightly by his bedside and he could recite by heart passages from Shakespeare and other poets. His grandson, Geoffrey Browne, recalls as a child being sat on FJ's knee and hearing *The Owl and the Pussycat* which FJ knew by heart. 'He spoke with an Irish accent: it was the Owl and the Poossycat that went to sea in a beautiful pea-green bort.'

Those of his letters that survive show that FJ was a great correspondent. There are family letters, letters while travelling – 'This afternoon we have seen lots of WHALES around the ship', for example, in a letter to his sister Sadie while aboard a rough crossing on the Cunard RMS *Aquitania* on 27 September 1934 en route to New York – and once he had moved to Australia he kept up a close correspondence with colleagues and others in England.

Many of John Browne's letters to his father and Grace from the 1950s and early '60s survive. These contain masses of family news, including work on the new edition of *Antenatal and Postnatal Care* that John wrote with his father, as well as occasional comments on national events (the Coronation and so forth) and items of obstetric interest (including the Queen's pregnancy with Prince Andrew). They also show that money was quite tight for John and that he had his father's capacity to work exceptionally long hours without complaining, though he does grumble at finding himself 'increasingly bogged down in administration and committees... there is far too much of this sort of work to do', a circumstance that has not entirely resolved itself in the NHS in the years hence.

There are many other letters from family and friends to FJ that survive but far fewer from him to others. However, what does survive is an extensive single volume war diary that FJ kept. He began it on Saturday 9 September 1939 writing:

'At 10.25 p.m. I begin this diary with the intention of recording the events of this momentous time as they affect me an ordinary British citizen. On Sunday last September 3rd at 11 a.m. war was declared by this country on Germany on account of her invasion of Poland which we had undertaken to defend.'

As is widely known, the first air raid siren went off shortly after war was declared and FJ records the event:

'At 11.30 the air raid system sounded. I was walking in the garden at the time and ran in telling everyone to put on their gas masks. We all went as fast as possible under the stairs and stayed there for some time, but hearing no shoot-ing nor any planes Henry and I came out to look round. Nothing was to be seen or heard and at 5 min. to 11² the 'all clear' signal went.'

It is difficult for today's generation to appreciate the effect that the war had on almost every sphere of life. Henry, reading modern languages at Pembroke College, Cambridge, volun-teered in the first few days at the university recruiting depot and shortly afterwards on 19 September celebrated his 21st birthday. Four days later he was ordered to report for his medical and FJ recorded, 'This means he will not return to Cambridge at begin-ning of this term as it is unlikely his calling up will be now long delayed. H. much more cheerful since'.

Amongst such family events the diary recalls the rapidly unfolding story on the international stage in the first twelve months of the war: the fall of Poland, Hitler's speeches, endless air raids, Russia's invasion of Finland, the fall of Denmark, Holland, Belgium and France, the 'epic' of Dunkirk and the first of Churchill's famous speeches. Henry's first solo flight was on September 3rd 1940 and his father sent him £1 'in celebration'. He got his 'wings' on December 6th and was home with pract-ically the whole family circle, only John missing, for Christmas.

With terrible prescience the diary entry for Christmas Day 1940 includes the underlined question 'What will have happened to the circle before.next Christmas?'.

The diary continues through to the end of the war recording both national and local events, including the mentioning of John Browne, Royal Air Force Volunteer Reserve, 'in a Despatch for distinguished service' and ends with brief, factual records of the surrender of Germany on May 7th 1945, the destruction of Hiroshima on August 8th and the surrender of Japan on August 15th. But the heart of the diary lies in 1941. On May 12th, the day before FJ records that Rudolf Hess landed his plane near Glasgow and was interned, came the terrible news that every parent in such a situation dreaded: Henry was reported missing. The diary entry reads:

'HENRY MISSING from Raid on Mannheim on Friday night last. At 6.15 p.m. today had a letter from No 57 Bomber Squadron, Dishforth, to say he "was second pilot of a crew that took off on Friday evening to attack a target at Mannheim. The operation was successfully carried out and a radio message was received on hour after leaving for their base. Since then nothing has been heard. A sweeping search has been carried out from dawn till near dusk on Saturday but nothing was found. It is thought they may have been picked up by an unknown ship or he may be (it is just possible he is) a prisoner of war".'

Two days later the diary entry includes:

'The worst of these days is the awful silence that has descended. Henry in his last letter said that he would 'write again at the weekend'. The letter would have arrived yesterday or today but there is nothing, nothing, nothing.'

FJ was told on May 18th by Henry's CO that he was 'confident they are prisoners of war' after a forced landing or a bale out but

FJ soon realised this was unlikely. On June 14th he records:

'Henry missing 5 weeks today and hope beginning to grow dim... Saturday nights are I think the most trying of the week. Henry used so often to come then on a few hours leave. Tonight he has not come and it is now 9.40. M has been weeping a little. A cold windy June night. Fire watching duty tonight 11–5 a.m.'

On June 17th they heard that Henry's bomber had been found with all the crew dead. However, even now the faint hope was not extinguished. There were only four bodies and it had been thought that the crew numbered five. It was possible that one of them had managed to bail out and it transpired that Henry would have been the first to jump once any order to bail out had been given.

Finally on 12 September, a week before what would have been his 23rd birthday, the family received official news from the Air Ministry to say that German official information reported that Henry had been killed in action and buried on May 11th 1941 at Eindhoven in Holland. The short diary entry for the day concludes 'How much we have all been hoping during the last four months we now realise'.

Notes

1 Peel, J. *The Gynaecological Visiting Society 1911–1971*. Dorchester: Dorset Press; 1992, p. 75.
2 Clearly a slip. '11' should be '12'.

Chapter Eight
The family

Among the documents preserved in the RANZCOG archives are many letters received by FJ Browne from his parents, siblings and children. Some of them were written forty or more years before his death and it is remarkable that he preserved them.

His father's (William Browne 1854–1944) letters, addressed 'My dear Frank' and signed 'Your affectionate father', are all carefully dated. On September 18th 1923 he writes about John in Australia (FJ's older brother) and says he does not want to give up the house and farm in Tullybogly 'as this would leave the girls without a home. You will understand it was not easy to say to John I don't want you to come home'. In a letter of May 11th 1926 he congratulates FJ on his appointment to UCH and writes 'words fail me to express what I feel when and since your letter has been read and reread: it is indeed great. I am sure you will feel the great responsibility resting on you as head of the Unit. But don't fear – you always succeed in whatever you undertake.'

Other letters express delight at Olive's and John's qualifying, report news of FJ's brothers and sisters, and describe work on the enlargement of the house and the work on the farm. He complains about rising taxes and poor returns, and sees little hope in the future of farming. There are also frequent references to rain and storms, interfering with the harvest. New apple and plum trees were obtained from McGredys in Portadown, as well as roses[1] and FJ advised him about adding fertiliser and manure when planting them out.

There are complaints about rail strikes interfering with dispatch of produce, and reports about local church affairs, the appointment of a new minister, parish council meetings, choir practices and even what hymns were sung at services. FJ's visits on the occasions of his examining in Belfast and Dublin are eagerly anticipated. (FJ used to visit his old home after examining in Belfast.) In a letter of March 11th 1935, he expresses his pleasure that *Antenatal and Postnatal Care* has been finished (the first edition appeared later that year) and says, 'Mother [i.e. FJ's grandmother] would have been pleased to know. Well perhaps she does know.'

His mother's (Sarah 1853–1933) letters are written in a similar affectionate style but are all undated. There is a charming letter of congratulation to FJ and Minnie on the birth of Eileen (1923) and pride in the achievements of Olive and John, her grand-children. There is much news of the family – health problems, and the state of the house, farm and garden.

Reading these letters shows the close relationship which existed between his parents and FJ who, although he had left home, still seemed to them to belong there.

This close family relationship is shown also in letters FJ pre-served from his three sisters, Matilda (Tilly), Sadie and Elizabeth.

Tilly, who never married, her fiancée having died in the influenza epidemic, became a hospital matron. She wrote a long and enthusiastic letter to FJ on May 7th 1926, congratulating him on becoming a 'real professor' but realising that he would be sad to leave Edinburgh. In a letter of June 2nd 1933 she describes a recent stay in Tullybogly where she nursed their mother, Sarah, who suffered from fatigue, breathlessness, cough and blueness of the lips and fingers. It sounds as if she was in heart failure, and she died that year. Later letters are written to FJ and Grace in Australia whom she visited in 1953 staying quite a long time. In 1959 she is congratulating Grace on becoming an FRCOG 'that makes three in the family' and being awarded the MBE.

Sadie also became a nurse (in those days careers for women were very limited) and also never married. Preserved letters from her to FJ date from 1932 to 1944 and demonstrate a very close brother–sister relationship. By 1933 their mother's health was declining and she was confined to bed most of the day. Sadie stayed at home to nurse her and care for her father and there are detailed clinical reports on her condition, as from nurse to doctor. She does not write about her mother's death and funeral: presumably FJ came back home at the time. There are many sad references to the death, funeral and grave site and to her father's depression. It is of interest that there are many scribbled lecture notes by FJ on the backs of Sadie's letters. He must have carried them around with him. In a letter of March 12th 1935, she congratulates FJ on having finished his book, 'My! Wouldn't mother have been proud?' and also writes 'Now about going to Vienna: are you serious when you talk of going by aeroplane? Father says he hopes you will have more sense!'

By 1943, the letters speak more and more of their father's misery and ill health: he was now 89 years old and in her letter of 5th January 1944, Sadie reports his passing away. Her letter of 27th January 1944 deserves quoting in full:

'As Mr Kennedy [the minister] said the words "Dust to dust, ashes to ashes", Harry who stood at the head of the grave stooped down and lifting some clay off mother's grave dropped it on top of the coffin. Elizabeth and I went up the day before yesterday to see the grave. The first glimpse made us very sad. Everything is very neat with the four wreaths. The snowdrops that he planted at the head of mother's grave are coming into bloom. I think I told you he is buried in the middle; one day he and I were there and he pointed to it with his stick and said this is where he wanted to lie. We think it is where his own father is buried and so had not been opened for 78 years. He was very proud of you and many a time talked about you.

No, I don't think I was anything wonderful. Father and I did not always agree, but we understood each other and were happy in our way... nothing can ever be the same again. I remember when mother died for a long time after it was so sad not having her about. It is strange how the days do go on. We have to eat and sleep and work until we too pass on. Father had to do it himself. Indeed I never thought he would survive mother so long.'

Poignant words indeed, that illustrate how close knit a family the Brownes were.

During his time at University College Hospital, FJ and Minnie lived at Heath Lodge in Bushey, near Watford. The house has been pulled down to make room for a modern development. FJ commuted by train to Marylebone Station in London, a 20-minute walk from UCH. He was a keen walker and did the journey on foot most days. However, there were considerable regrets about his having to move to London, leaving the Edinburgh he loved, with his daily walk from home to hospital.

They had four children. Olive Mildred, the oldest, was born in Abertillery in 1909. After attending school at Craigmont School in Edinburgh, she studied medicine at Edinburgh University, where she lived in Masson Hall, and qualified in 1934. As a student, one of her memories was seeing newborn babies attended to on brown paper on kitchen tables.

Olive held a number of junior appointments and contemplated becoming an anaesthetist. However, she had to resign (such were the rules in those days) from an appointment in an LCC Hospital in London when she got married and had children. Later she specialised in medical gynaecology with special interests in adolescent and psychosexual problems and ultimately became Consultant to the University Health Service in the new University of Surrey. She married John Vernon Hurford, qualified in Belfast, a Fellow of the Royal College of Physicians, who was a chest physician and became Medical Superintendent of King George V Sanatorium near Godalming. They had two children, Ann, born in 1940, who never married and does not remember her grandparents well, and David, born in 1944, who lives in Devon and has been particularly helpful with stories and reminiscences of his grandfather.

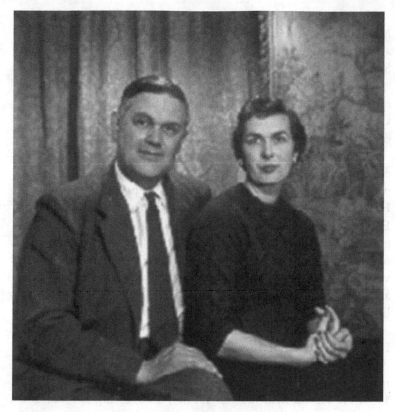

Olive and John Hurford

Olive had a close relationship with her father and there are, in the records, letters they exchanged and even a tape of a telephone conversation with her father and Grace when they lived in Australia.

She was an accomplished pianist and especially skilled at improvisation and adapting the music of Gilbert and Sullivan to hospital pantomime scripts. She was a renowned and creative cook with particular leanings to French cuisine. Her hobbies, apart from music, were the arts and theatre, and she took up painting in later life.

She was a Fellow (like her father) of the Royal Society of Medicine and the Eugenics Society and lectured widely on abortion, the generation gap, the NHS and the affluent society. She died in 1991.

FJ preserved many of her letters which date from her time as a medical student in Edinburgh in 1930 until just before his death. Olive addresses her father as 'Dada'. There are detailed accounts of examinations, graduation ceremony and life as a resident.

Her later letters to Australia are full of family news and reveal close contacts with John and Eileen and their families. The possibility of FJ and Grace's return to England is discussed. Heath Lodge was let, but still belonged to FJ. They did visit England in 1955 after which Olive wrote, 'It was a wrench to say good-bye, though I know that travel in itself is a wonderful thing for you to be able to do. But you must know that we are all very very fond of you and don't entirely appreciate the fact that you are so far away'. Just like John, she hoped they would return to live in England: however, this was not to be.

The second child, and first son, was John Campbell McClure Browne, also born in Abertillery, in 1912.

He went to school at the Edinburgh Academy and studied medicine at University College Hospital, London, qualifying in 1937. He served with the Royal Air Force during the war and was twice mentioned in despatches. He specialised in obstetrics and gynaecology and worked under James Young at Hammersmith Hospital and Robert Kellar in Edinburgh. He was appointed Professor at the Postgraduate Medical School and Director of the Institute of Obstetrics and Gynaecology in 1952.

Like his father, he was an excellent clinician and great teacher and in particular became advisor and mentor to countless postgraduates from home and abroad. He collaborated with FJ on *Antenatal and Postnatal Care* (the last edition of which he edited with Geoffrey Dixon) and was co-author of *Postgraduate Obstetrics and Gynaecology*. His research was mainly on placental circulation and post-maturity. He was a member of many committees at national and international level and was appointed CBE in 1975. He retired in 1977 and sadly died the following year. He was survived by his wife, Veronica, and their son, Geoffrey (born 1946) who became a musician, playing the oboe and English horn. He has written on these and teaches at the Royal Academy of Music. He has been of particular help in compiling this biography. Their daughter, Mary, was born after FJ migrated to Australia and so did not know her grandfather.

There is, among the Australian archives, an almost complete file of the letters John wrote about fortnightly to his father in Sydney. They are a unique combination of the personal and the professional. They are addressed to 'dear FJ and Grace' and usually terminate 'with love from us all'. On a personal level, John and Veronica, as well as Eileen, lived at Heath Lodge for some time after the departure of FJ and Grace. The letters speak of the house, redecoration, garden, insurance and other relevant matters. They are full of Geoffrey's progress, his chicken pox, his schools and interest in music and, at the age of seven, his 'growing to be a splendid boy and good company'. There are problems with au pairs, the hazards of electric lawn mowers, and even the dog: 'Our corgi had 6 puppies (father a Dalmatian!). Obstructed labour. All breech presentations. Only one survived, delivered by me with ovum forceps under chloroform.' There are thanks for food parcels (rationing was still enforced in the early 1950s), gifts of wine, postal orders for Geoffrey. Holidays were described and, above all, the tight financial situation which was typical of a whole-time academic at the time. Veronica had a second child, Mary, in 1953, delivered by caesarean section by Will Nixon (FJ's successor as Professor at UCH) and he was 'kindness personified'. John got his first cine-camera and sent movies of the children to their grandparents in Australia. There are even items of gossip: 'The Queen is pregnant and Peel is looking after her' and 'went to a party at GA's [VB Greene-Armytage] last night – endless people asking after you' and 'when does he return?'

The close ties between father and son are clearly illustrated by this correspondence. Throughout there is the hope that FJ and

Grace would return to England: 'Delighted that you are ward teaching at the North Shore [Hospital] and only wish you were doing the same here. If you do decide to stay, I will understand, but if you return, you know how glad we shall be'.

On the professional level, the correspondence is most revealing. There are long discussions on the results of trial labour (Gibberd's views are strongly criticised), the treatment of carcinoma of the body of the uterus, the aetiology of eclampsia and other gynaecological problems. John undertook the final revision of *Antenatal and Postnatal Care* and *Postgraduate Obstetrics and Gynaecology* and there are detailed discussions about minutiae, as well as consideration of advances in technique and treatment. John's own research, mainly on placental blood flow, is discussed at length and he expresses his frustration that with endless clinical work, teaching, administration, speaking at meetings, entertaining visitors and attending congresses, he has too little time to pursue his own research interests. He comments on his colleagues – Charles Read and Robin Murdoch with whom he obviously has excellent relations and, amongst others, mentions, in 1952, a newly appointed assistant, Ian Donald who 'is shaping well'.[2]

John saw his father on a tour of Australia in 1962, a year before FJ's death.

The third child, Henry Gallaugher Browne, was born in Abertillery on September 19th, 1918, and christened in memory of his mother's brother, Henry Gallaugher, who served with the Royal Inniskilling Fusiliers and was killed in the First World War, having been awarded the Distinguished Service Order for 'conspicuous gallantry in action'. After initial schooling in Edinburgh and London, Henry went to Epsom College and boarded at Carr House from 1932 to 1937. In his school days, he excelled more at shooting at Bisley than in academic work. An exchange of letters between his house-master and FJ comments on his charm of manner and even temper (23 January 1935). He did better in English, French and Latin than in mathematics (despite extra tuition), physics, chemistry and biology, and this is borne out by his being in the

'V! Lit' form in his last year. He was a member of the OTC (Officers' Training Corps), but even at this stage was more interested in joining the Royal Air Force.

Henry's letters home from school are typical of those written by any boarding school boy. There are references to masters, other boys, food, a stay in the sanatorium for mumps, joy at receiving postal orders and parcels of biscuits and chocolates, moans about work and examinations, and long discussions about whether to go to camp or not. He was an acute observer, able to put his views and experiences into words in a highly developed and descriptive manner. This is clearly illustrated by the following quotation in a letter dated May 31st (no year stated):

> 'I am sure I am doing much better at Maths than I have ever done before. Mr Raymond simply beats me if I make even a slightly careless slip. I can't help laughing till I nearly cry when he says 'Bend over Browne'. He makes me absolutely grasp my toes and then brings down the beastly pointer or his little devil of an ebony ruler. He's quite humorous about it, at least so far.
>
> I think he likes beating. He takes a terribly long time over each lash, and laughs and says I am not touching my toes. He gets precisely the same spot each time too, however much you twist'.

A clearer description of a sadistic master could not have been written: at least beating and 'fagging' to which he also refers, have been abolished in British public schools.

Henry passed his 'Matric' examination, and proceeded to become a member of Pembroke College, Cambridge, where he was formally admitted to the University on November 2nd 1938. In his application form he put '? consular service' as his proposed profession. He must have done reasonably well because in his first term, Michaelmas 1938, he was excused from taking all three parts of the 'Previous' examination. He read for the Medieval and Modern Language Tripos and was resident in the university for two years – the first lodging at 1 Fitzwilliam Street and the second at 8 Downing Street, both adjacent to the college. Rowing and tennis occupied most of his spare time and he was in his college's first boat. He used to visit John, his older brother, who was stationed nearby. Veronica was praised for her cooking and Henry used to borrow John's car.

Henry left Cambridge at the end of Easter Term 1940 and, like his brother, joined the Royal Air Force. On July 16th 1941 he was 'allowed' the three remaining terms to complete a degree. This meant he was eligible to graduate even though he had not been in residence for the period usually required to gain a degree. Such dispensation was common during the war and he was awarded a posthumous degree in January 1942.

After training, which took a year, he became a sergeant pilot in 51 Squadron of the Royal Air Force Volunteer Reserve. He was shot down, in what must have been one of his first missions, over Holland, returning from a bombing raid over Germany, on May 10th 1941 He was buried in the General Cemetery of Eindhoven, a small town in East Holland, near the German frontier. About 700 British casualties have their final resting place here: most of them were members of the RAF, but there are also some members of the land forces who died there between September 1944 and May 1945.

It was a long time before his parents knew of his fate and FJ in his wartime diaries records their distress. They, together with Eileen, visited the grave after the war. There is a note in a letter of Olive's to FJ (May 1955) that she had been to Heath Lodge, which was let during FJ's absence 'and I also took into my charge (and will look after most carefully) a box containing Henry's letters and a school photograph of the cricket team with Henry in it. Really I could not bear to see them just stored.'

Eileen, the youngest, was also born in Edinburgh, in 1923. After leaving school, she studied at the Royal College of Music and then briefly taught music at Overstone School in Northampton. During the war she worked in a munitions factory in Watford.

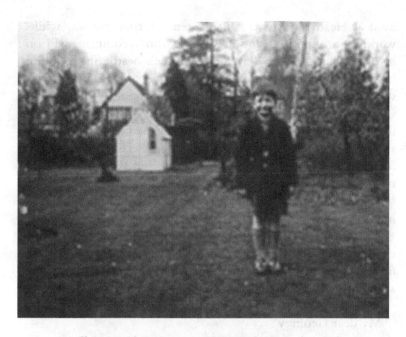

Geoffrey McClure Browne, FJ's grandson, in the garden
at Heath Lodge

She joined the BBC in 1946 as a programme assistant and
became best known as an early presenter of *Listen with Mother*.
She also took part in and directed many other productions. After
an unhappy first marriage, in which she had a 'bad' miscarriage,
she married Robert Mitchell, a Kent farmer and fruit grower.
They had two children, Robert and Lydia. Her skills at music
and storytelling never left her and were much appreciated by her
grandchildren. She died in 1999. She had always been very close
to her father.

Her letters are most affectionate, starting 'My dearest Dada'
and finishing with 'my dear love to you'. There are typical
schoolgirl letters about music and dancing lessons, girl guides,
fierce headmistresses, tennis, pets, rehearsals for *The Magic Flute*
and listening to Beethoven sonatas on the gramophone. She

lived at Heath Lodge with her parents during the war whilst working in munitions, and it was she who accompanied FJ on his Australian tour in 1950 after Minnie's death. She left him here and flew back home: in those days a very long journey with stops brilliantly described in Darwin, Singapore, Bombay and Cairo. Her later letters describe her work at the BBC, singing in the Bach Choir, life at Burnham and her passion for gardening about which she became very knowledgeable. She wrote to her father at length after the birth of John and Veronica's second child, Mary, and after describing the baby, mentions Geoffrey who 'is a fine sturdy boy and gets better looking each time I see him'.

There remain few letters from FJ to his children and grand-children. One of the most poignant, written on August 21st 1956 from Australia to his grandson, Geoffrey, aged ten at the time, accompanied a Bible which had belonged to FJ's son, Henry:

My dear Geoffrey

This Bible, as you will see from the front page, was given to your uncle Henry by Walter Gale. Henry was a member of the Crusaders, a religious youth group in Watford Parish Church, of which Walter Gale was the leader. Like Henry he was, I think, killed in the war.

I value the little Bible very much, and I am sure you will too. I am sure Henry would like you to have it.

Your affectionate Grandfather,
FJ Browne

Notes

1 McGredys – still one of the world's best rose growers – have emigrated from Northern Ireland to New Zealand.

2 Ian Donald revolutionised obstetrics by the application, development and use of ultrasound. He became Professor of Obstetrics and Gynaecology in Glasgow and must rank as one of the (if not the) most important figures of the specialty in the second half of the 20th century.

Chapter Nine
Interregnum

FJ retired from his Chair at UCH in 1946, having reached the age of 67. It is a great shock, both physical and mental, for one who has been so active in his profession, which he had made his life, to be faced suddenly with compulsory idleness.

But he had other causes for a deep depression.

Both he and Minnie were grieving at Henry's death, full details of which did not reach them until the end of the war. The loss of a dearly loved son is hard to bear. In addition Minnie's health was deteriorating and she became weaker and eventually died at home on August 22nd 1948, at the age of 64 years. The death certificate gives (a) carcinomatosis, (b) carcinoma of the lung as causes of death.

But idleness and depression were concepts foreign to FJ. Instead of giving way, he responded to these tragic circumstances in the way one would have expected him to: he immersed himself in work.

He started work as an Honorary Senior Lecturer at the Institute of Obstetrics and Gynaecology, based in the Postgraduate Medical School at Hammersmith Hospital in London. His main contributions here were the weekly ward rounds he held for teaching. Norman Morris[1] remembers these 'grand rounds' which involved all the gynaecologists as well as the pathologists:

'There was one famous morning when he was there together with Charles Read, James Young, and of course

John McClure Browne. It was a wonderful morning and the discussion was very lively... I had a funny feeling at this meeting that I would never hear this kind of debate again and it sadly became true in the next month or so when Charles Read died quite suddenly.'

FJ also started courses of formal teaching and lectures for post-graduates, most of whom were preparing for the examination for membership of the Royal College. They were held at the Soho Hospital for Women and at the City of London Maternity Hospital. These soon became immensely popular and attracted students from home and abroad. Elliot Philipp attended one such course and remembers vividly 'the excellence of the teaching, the ability to communicate and to present the subject clearly. He spoke slowly and precisely and presented much material which had not yet been published and would have been difficult to find elsewhere.'

These lectures formed the basis for FJ's next book, *Postgraduate Obstetrics and Gynaecology*, first published in 1950 and a tremendous achievement of single authorship. The second edition in 1955 appeared under joint authorship with his son, Professor McClure Browne. It consists of some 45 chapters, totalling nearly 700 pages and deals with subjects at a more advanced level than *Antenatal and Postnatal Care*: the latter having been aimed at medical students and general practitioners whilst this volume was intended for budding specialists. In the Preface to the first edition FJ states his philosophy of teaching: 'The aim of the teacher should be, I think, to know the literature as far as he can, to filter it through his mind and give his conclusions, right or wrong. In short to present the subject as he sees it in the light of his reading, thinking and personal experience.' Both this volume and the previously published *Antenatal and Postnatal Care* were at that time unique in English obstetric literature and it is impossible to understate the influence they had as virtually compulsory reading for those in training to undertake obstetrics or to become specialists.

In 1950, FJ, by now 71 years old and very much an 'elderly statesman' in the world of obstetrics, was awarded a travelling scholarship by the Royal College and at the invitation of the King George VI and Queen Elizabeth Fund for Mothers and Babies visited Australia and New Zealand. On the long outward boat journey he was accompanied by his daughter, Eileen. In the course of the tour, he visited many centres of excellence throughout Australia and New Zealand and also seized the opportunity to establish communication with members of the family who had settled there. His lectures and clinical demonstrations were enthusiastically received.

In Sydney, FJ was shown around by Dr Grace Cuthbert, then 50 years old, a well known local obstetrician and Director of Maternal and Baby Welfare in the Department of Health of New South Wales. As she was to become FJ's second wife, it is appropriate at this stage to say something of her background and career.

Grace was born in 1900 in Port Glasgow in Scotland, the fifth and youngest child of Captain and Mrs John Cuthbert. Her father was a merchant sailor and the first ship he commanded was engaged in the frozen mutton trade between New Zealand and England. Grace's mother was a primary school headmistress, highly accomplished and well educated who lived until 1937 and kept in close contact with members of the family in Scotland after she had settled in Australia. In 1901, Captain Cuthbert took up an appointment as chief marine surveyor for a group of insurance companies, and this is when the whole family moved to Sydney. The family were strong Presbyterians.

Grace went to school in Sydney. At the outbreak of the 1914 war, her three brothers went to do war service in England. One of them was killed. In 1918, she started to study medicine at Sydney University and, after qualifying, became interested in obstetrics and the care of the newborn. After wide experience as a resident and in practice, she was appointed to her present post in 1937. 'We struggled hard to reduce the maternal and infant mortality rates.' She travelled abroad extensively and in 1950 was awarded a travelling fellowship by the World Health Organ-

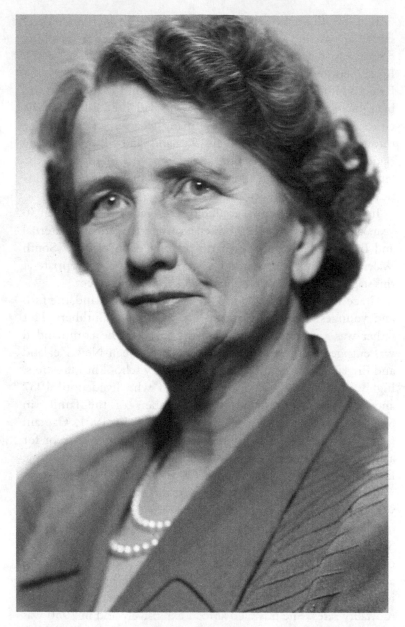

Dr Grace Cuthbert

ization. She tells how the publication of FJ's *Antenatal and Postnatal Care* in 1935 'fulfilled all my requirements for up-to-date guidance in the antenatal supervision of my patients' and how intensely subsequent editions were studied.

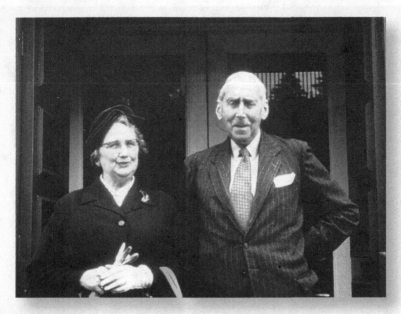

FJ and Grace after their wedding in 1951

Grace met FJ in Sydney in 1950; later that year she travelled overseas to North America, Scandinavia, France and Britain, where she saw FJ again in London. The relationship developed rapidly and they were married in February 1951 in the Crown Court National Church of Scotland in London. John McClure was best man and Elizabeth and Margaret, Grace's nieces, were bridesmaids.

Note

1   Later Professor at Charing Cross Hospital and Dean of the Medical Faculty, University of London.

Chapter Ten

Australia

When FJ and Grace returned to Australia in 1951, no firm decision had been made about where they were going to live permanently. Grace felt honour bound to resume her work as Director of the New South Wales Maternal and Baby Welfare Department: after all, it had been this position which had led to her being offered the WHO Fellowship. Grace's appointment entailed much travelling and taking part in conferences in Australia. During these separations, she wrote many letters to FJ, unfortunately all undated. They show clearly the depth of love of their relationship: 'Dearest, Still seems so odd without you – I hope you are missing me. It would be lovely to have you here – you seem such a long way away. All my love – Your Grace'.

Initially, they decided not to sell Heath Lodge, FJ's London home. His furniture and belongings remained there and indeed he and Grace stayed there for some weeks after the wedding. Then the house was used by FJ's children, and later it was let. The children's letters to FJ express their wishes and hope that they would eventually return to settle in England.

FJ is said to have remarked that London was not big enough to hold two Professors Browne, an apocryphal story which is out of character and unlikely to have been true. More likely he was influenced by the enthusiastic welcome he received from the Australian obstetric community. He was appointed to the consultant staff of three distinguished hospitals: the Royal North

Shore Hospital and the Royal Hospital for Women and also to the Royal Newcastle Hospital. He took part in staff conferences, conducted teaching ward rounds and taught both undergraduates and postgraduates This involved much travelling for a man of his age. Inevitably he became well known as a teacher and his ward rounds were particularly well attended. His contributions to staff conferences with his friendly, unassuming manner combined with wide knowledge and a highly critical approach, were much appreciated.

Ian Cope records that he was 'greatly inspired by his searching questions on histopathology and clinical management and encouraged by him to undertake work which eventually led to my MD'. The welcome extended beyond hospital work. Australians displayed their superb hospitality and made him very welcome, both socially and professionally.

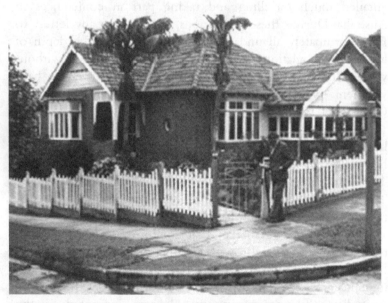

FJ outside his home in the Sydney suburb of Wollstonecraft

The result is that they bought a house in 1953 and moved into 2 Gillies Street, in Wollstonecraft, a suburb of Sydney on June 19th 1953. It was to be FJ's last home. The house is still standing, a pleasant family house in an agreeable neighbourhood, with a spacious garden.

Whilst Grace continued in her post, FJ was fully occupied, not only with teaching, but also with new editions of his books and the writing of scientific articles and reviews, for which he was in great demand. He could read German (though his pronunciation was said to be rather strange). He was an avid reader and developments in obstetric practice were proceeding so rapidly that just 'keeping up to date' was a major task. What spare time remained was devoted to gardening and, dressed like any old gardener, he tended his plants. He was particularly keen on growing carnations and roses. When they moved in, a neighbour told FJ that 'you can't grow roses in Wollstonecraft'. FJ had great pleasure in proving him wrong.

Their lives were so busy that they welcomed a prolonged visit from Tilly who helped with running the household. FJ and Grace were considered a highly talented couple and were widely respected and loved. They entertained frequently and widely, not only their Australian friends and colleagues, but also visitors from Britain. As Theobald[1] said, 'No visiting obstetrician left Sydney without paying court to FJ'.

Grace was an excellent cook and FJ a generous host who entertained his guests with recitals from Shakespeare and other of his favourite writers and poets. He always insisted on doing the washing-up by himself, even after a full table, and recited Gray's Elegy while doing it.

Chris Cuthbert, Grace's nephew, recounts how he was there at dinner when Grace was awarded the MBE (her brother, a distinguished ENT surgeon in Perth was an OBE) and 'FJ was bristling away at his end of the table 'Absolute disgrace, absolute disgrace. She should have sent it back. I told her she should have been a Dame!'.

The marriage turned out to be a time of happiness and fulfilment. They were united not only by their professional interests; there was also a deep love and understanding. FJ's calm and stability were to be the perfect foil to Grace's highly strung temperament. A streak of romanticism is shown in a letter found after Grace's death, dated 25 December 1957 which reads:

'To Grace with love.

> Then in these thoughts myself almost despising,
> Haply I think on thee and then my state,
> Like to the lark at break of day arising
> From sullen earth sings hymns at Heaven's Gate.
> So thy sweet love remembered all things brings
> And then I would not change my state with Kings.'

These are in fact the last six lines of Shakespeare's 29th sonnet. The accepted version of the last two lines is:

> 'For thy sweet love remembered such wealth brings
> That then I scorn to change my state with kings.'

The different version shows that the lines were quoted from memory – a remarkable feat for a man of 79 years.

The regard in which FJ was held by his Australian colleagues is demonstrated by the fact that after his death the New South Wales State Committee and the Australian College created a commemorative medal, the FJ Browne medal, to be awarded to a Member or a Fellow of not more than five years standing for the most outstanding scientific contribution. In 1971 it was decided that the medal should in future go to the candidate obtaining the highest marks in the second part of the MRCOG examination held in Australia. The list of names of the recipients since the inauguration of the medal in 1964 reads like a roll of honour with many distinguished doctors who have

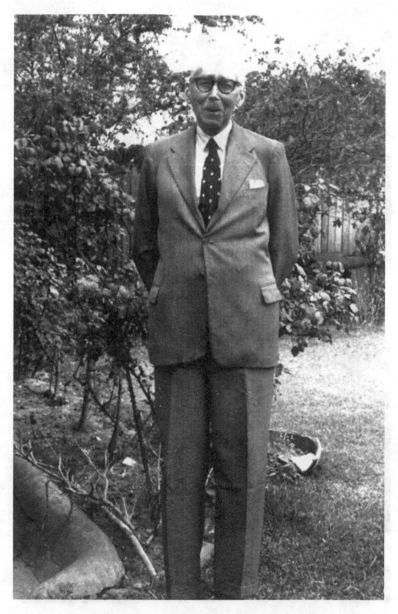

FJ, photographed by Grace in the back garden, December 1958

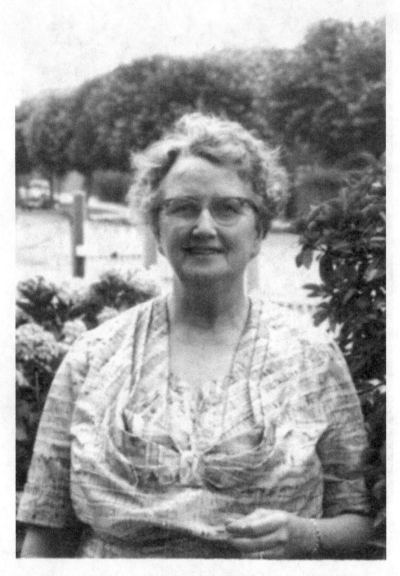

Grace, taken by FJ in the front garden, December 1958

subsequently made important contributions to the practice of, and research in, obstetrics and gynaecology.

FJ's health gradually declined. When he was awarded the Blair–Bell Medal of the Royal Society of Medicine in 1960, he felt too frail to attend the ceremony in London. At the age of 83 years he was admitted to the Royal North Shore Hospital where he stayed for some months. He died at his home on August 17th 1963. 'Grace had stretched every nerve to get him better, but alas, without success. At the end he just wanted to go and said so several times.'

The death certificate gives pulmonary embolism and Hodgkin's disease as the causes of death. He was cremated and the ashes interred at Waverley Cemetery, a well known landmark on the coast of Sydney.

Note

1   GW Theobald, formerly Professor of Obstetrics and Gynaecology, Bangkok, later consultant in Bradford.

Chapter Eleven

Epilogue

When FJ died in August 1963, Grace was distraught with grief. Later she wrote of his intellectual attainments and his gentle, loving kindness, of 'the enormous influence he had on me during 13 years of marriage', of his great inspiration and his continual encouragement and expert advice to her and her department. She records in particular his tremendous contribution as a member of the Special Committee investigating Maternal Mortality.[1]

Grace returned to work 'as he would have wished' as Director of the Maternal and Baby Welfare Department of New South Wales until her retirement in 1965. She also served on many other related committees and became President of the Australian Federation of University Women and of that of Medical Women. She was Vice President of he Medical Women's International Association. At the same time she kept up close relations with FJ's families in England and Ireland and visited them on regular trips. As recorded in an earlier chapter, she also visited FJ's old school in Londonderry and made a gift of a portrait of FJ, new furnishings and a commemorative plaque. Eventually she took up residence at the Northaven Retirement Village where she died at the age of 88 years on December 17th 1988. The death certificate gives pneumonia and septicaemia secondary to metastatic bowel cancer as cause of death.

Following FJ's death, very many eloquent obituaries appeared in the medical press in testimony of his great achievements,

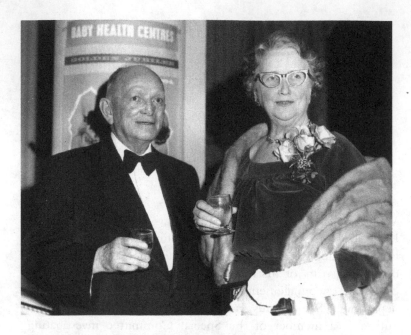

Grace, with the Health Minister, W Sheehan, at the reception in her
honour, held on 4 December 1964

demonstrating the universal respect and affection he inspired in
colleagues and friends.

In the *British Medical Journal* Professor WCW Nixon, his
successor at University College Hospital, describes his dyna-
mic personality and the stardom he achieved at a time when
it was still possible for an individual to influence ideas and
practice.[2]

GW Theobald wrote of his dour and shrewd character and
ends with 'we shall not see his like again'. Professor Chassar Moir
writes of him as his much loved old chief, a teacher with a
mission to instruct and instinctive power to train others in
logical thought and lucid writing. John Sophian speaks of his
powerful influence in the profession and above all his true
kindness.

In *The Lancet,* Gladys Dodds writes of his ability to think, talk and teach.[3] 'He was a hard worker' and taught his assistants to make accurate observations and write detailed notes.

Leslie Williams comments on his extensive knowledge, his popularity and his ability as a 'natural teacher'. Tim Flew, another of his former assistants, wrote in the *Journal of Obstetrics and Gynaecology of the British Commonwealth* of his personality and appearance: 'he was one of the best teachers of undergraduates that there has ever been'.[4] His systemic lectures were memorable and his ward rounds packed. He himself was 'a most sympathetic and understanding person'.

Professor Robert Kellar of Edinburgh, another former assistant, addressed the Council of the RCOG and described his influence on the teaching and practice of obstetrics as unique throughout the whole Commonwealth: 'here we had a really great clinician teacher at his best. The careful accurate history, the meticulous examination and reasoned discussion were the essential ingredients of his teaching'.

Similar tributes were paid to FJ in the Australian journals by Ian Monk of the North Shore Hospital, Sydney, and by Dr James Isbister, in a penetrating review of his life and work, in the *Medical Journal of Australia.*[5] Twenty-four years after FJ's death, Ian Cope presented a paper: 'FJ Browne and his influence on Australian obstetrics' at the 75th anniversary celebration of antenatal care at the Royal Hospital for Women, Sydney.[6] This is the most complete and satisfactory account of FJ's life and work, ending with the 13 years he spent in Sydney. He describes 'the feeling of friendship FJ radiated, his animated conversation, his pungent yet kindly wit and the unexpected remark often uttered in a light-hearted off-hand manner, but which when later considered was more penetrating and carried a deeper truth than was at first apparent'.

Of all the many tributes, the most poignant is that delivered by Chassar Moir at the 107th meeting of the Gynaecological Visiting Society. He writes with profound insight into the problems FJ and his family had faced in moving from Wales to

Edinburgh. It was at this time, as a house surgeon at the Simpson Memorial Hospital, that he first met FJ. He describes how the Obstetric Unit became a centre of attraction to visitors from near and far and later how FJ himself became the acknowledged doyen of the Australian obstetric community.

'Of Francis Browne the man, I find it difficult to speak, for he was very dear to me. Eccentric he was, and disconcertingly so with unpredictable action and words. Forgetful too, as becomes all true professors. An unprecedented honour was bestowed on him when he was elected to Honorary Membership of the GVS. I can think of no one in his time who was more honest of purpose or kind of heart.'

What remains to be said of this man who never stopped working and whose extraordinary life encompassed living in Northern Ireland, Aberdeen, a mining town in a Welsh valley, Edinburgh, University College Hospital and New South Wales? – certainly the regard with which he has been and is still held as a great obstetrician, an outstanding teacher and a writer with an enduring legacy; and equally the affection his personality inspired in his family and friends, colleagues and pupils.

When FJ first joined Ballantyne's team in Edinburgh, the maternal mortality rate was about 4.5 deaths per thousand deliveries and the stillbirth rate was over fifty per thousand births. By the time he left UCH, the corresponding figures were around 0.6 per thousand and forty per thousand. Today the maternal mortality is about 0.1 per thousand and the perinatal mortality (a new concept including stillbirths and first week neonatal deaths) is less than ten per thousand.

Ballantyne's original concept that maternal morbidity and mortality, as well as the stillbirth rate, could be reduced by better antenatal care inspired FJ and his contemporaries to apply his precepts to the whole field of obstetrics. Improvements in the maternity services and the results obtained, in the second half of the 20th century, stem from many factors. Improved antenatal care, greater attention to hygiene and the avoidance of sepsis, better anaesthetic techniques, the availability of blood transfusion, the introduction first of sulphonamides, later antibiotics and the reduction of deaths from abortion, following the introduction of the Abortion Act, have been of primary significance. The abolition of prolonged labour, avoidance of difficult vaginal deliveries and routine use of oxytocics have played a great role. Obstetricians have been the first to introduce regular audit into their work. Above all, the creation of the Royal College of Obstetricians and Gynaecologists has set standards of the utmost importance for the development of maternity services. It was the Foundation Fellows, of whom FJ was one, who made such developments possible.

Better training of medical students and midwives, avoidance of sepsis and the development of new obstetric techniques – conservative in some cases, radical in others, were essential tools. Ballantyne and Browne led the way in introducing the necessary changes, based on meticulous care of the pregnant woman and preventing or at least anticipating many of the mishaps to which she is subject.

Antenatal care today is different from that of fifty years ago. Personnel and techniques have changed; the approach to the individual woman has become more personal and flexible. The importance of calculating risk and means to reduce it have become important aspects of antenatal care. Vaccination against rubella and the administration of folic acid in the first trimester of pregnancy are preventing many fetal abnormalities.

The widespread use of ultrasound, resulting from the work of Ian Donald, has revolutionised obstetric practice. The enormous reduction in maternal mortality has focused attention more and more on the survival and wellbeing of the baby. Antenatal diagnosis of fetal abnormalities, first by amniocentesis, and later with the help of ultrasound and biochemical markers has been the most important innovation. The 1967 Abortion Act familiarised obstetricians with the practice of amniocentesis (previously only performed in the management of rhesus incompatibility) for second trimester terminations.[7] Amniocentesis resulted in the development of a whole new science not only of antenatal diagnosis, but also pre-implantation diagnosis. This has led to fetal surgery in some cases and pregnancy termination in others. Cynics may say that the latter merely transposes figures from the perinatal mortality to the abortion statistics. But ask parents who have struggled with the arduous and heartbreaking task of caring for an abnormal child and most will support such action. Antenatal care has indeed become 'personalised'. Techniques of antenatal care may have changed, but they still have as their object a safe and satisfactory result for mother and baby.

Greatness is a rare human quality. It consists of vision, achievement and persistence: abilities not given to many. It requires clarity of thought and skills of leadership. If combined with kindness, consideration and absence of malignity, it becomes particularly special. In every walk of life there exist some men and women who attain such heights. Francis Browne was one who did and who had a lasting influence on those of us who practise the same specialty and hope that our exertions pass benefits on to women.

Notes

1　Browne, GC. *Women Physicians of the World*. London: Hemisphere Publishing; 1978, pp. 187–197.
2　British Medical Journal 1963: 31 August.
3　*Lancet* 1963; 31 August 31:471.
4　Journal of Obstetrics and Gynaecology of the British Commonwealth 1963;70:108–182.
5　*Medical Journal of Australia* 1963; 14 December:1002.
6　Australia and New Zealand Journal of Obstetrics and Gynaecology 1988;28:85–89.
7　Amniocentesis, first introduced in the UK by Butler and Reiss in 1970 for the antenatal diagnosis of Down syndrome, enabled embryologists to grow amniotic fetal cells in culture and study their chromosome composition.

Francis James Browne (1879–1963): A Bibliography

Books

Browne FJ (1926) *Advice to the Expectant Mother on the Care of Her Health*. Livingstone, Edinburgh

Browne FJ (1928) *ibid* 2nd edn

Browne FJ (1934) *ibid* 3rd edn

Browne FJ (1938) *ibid* 4th edn

Browne FJ (1940) *Advice to the Expectant Mother on the Care of Her Health and That of Her Child*. 5th edn

Browne FJ (1942) *ibid* 6th edn

Browne FJ (1944) *ibid* 7th edn

Browne FJ (1947) *ibid* 8th edn

Browne FJ (1951) *ibid* 9th edn

Browne FJ (1953) *ibid* 10th edn. Livingstone, Edinburgh and London

Browne FJ; Browne JCM (1957) *ibid* 11th edn

Browne FJ; Browne JCM (1962) *Advice to the Expectant Mother on the Care of Her Health and That of Her Child. Section on Feeding and Care of the Baby By JPM Tizard*. 12th edn

Browne FJ; Browne JCM (1966) *ibid* 13th edn

A fourteenth edition appeared in 1973, edited by JCM Browne.

Browne FJ (1935) *Antenatal and Postnatal Care*. Churchill, London

Browne FJ (1937) *ibid* 2nd edn

Browne FJ (1939) *ibid* 3rd edn

Browne FJ (1942) *ibid* 4th edn

Browne FJ (1944) *ibid* 5th edn

Browne FJ (1946) *ibid* 6th edn

Browne FJ (1951) *ibid* 7th edn

Browne FJ; Browne JCM (1955) *ibid* 8th edn

Browne FJ; Browne JCM (1960) *ibid* 9th edn

Subsequent editions are entitled *Browne's Antenatal Care*. A tenth edition appeared in 1970 under the joint editorship of JCM Browne and G Dixon, who together edited an eleventh and final edition in 1978.

Translations appeared in Chinese (1949), Spanish (1951) and Turkish (1963).

Browne FJ (1937) *Obstetric Technique: Methods in Use in the Obstetric Unit, University College Hospital, London*. Wilding & Son Ltd, Shrewsbury.

Browne FJ (1940) *ibid* 2nd edn

Browne FJ (1943) *ibid* 3rd edn

Browne FJ (1945) *ibid* 4th edn

Browne FJ (1948) *ibid* 5th edn

Browne FJ (1950) *Postgraduate Obstetrics and Gynaecology*. Butterworth, London.

Browne FJ; Browne JCM (1955) *ibid* 2nd edn

Browne FJ; Browne JCM (1964) *ibid* 3rd edn

A fourth edition appeared in 1973, edited by JC M Browne.

Hammond J; Browne FJ; Wolstenholme GEW, editors (1950) *Toxaemias of Pregnancy: Human and Veterinary*. Ciba Foundation Symposium. Churchill, London.

Contributions to books and journals

1912

Browne FJ; Mackenzie JR. The etiology and treatment of miner's nystagmus: with a review of 100 cases. *British Medical Journal* 1912;2:837–40.

1920

Browne FJ. On the histology of hydatidiform mole in its relation to prognosis. *Transactions of the Obstetrical Society of Edinburgh* 1919–1920;XL:26–41.

Ballantyne JW, Browne FJ. The colour scheme in pregnancy. *Transactions of the Obstetrical Society of Edinburgh* 1919–1920;XL:74–89.

Browne FJ. The anencephalic syndrome in its relation to apituitarism. *Edinburgh Medical Journal* 1920;New Series XXV:296–307.

Browne FJ. After-results from the Edinburgh antenatal clinic. *International Clinics* 1920;2:(Thirtieth series) 280–92.

1921

Browne FJ. Syphilis in the newborn. An investigation into the pathology of 21 cases. *Journal of Obstetrics and Gynaecology of the British Empire* 1921;28:153–89.

Browne FJ; Stillbirth: its causes, pathology and prevention. *British Medical Journal* 1921;2:140–45.

Browne FJ. Still-birth: its causes, pathology and prevention. *Edinburgh Medical Journal* 1921;New Series XXVII:153–66; 199–211; 286-296.

Browne FJ. Still-birth: its causes, pathology and prevention. *Transactions of the Edinburgh Obstetrical Society* 1920–1921;XLI:82–133.

Johnstone RW; Browne FJ Case of double congenital hydronephrosis. *Transactions of the Edinburgh Obstetrical Society* 1920–1921 XLI 29–35.

[Browne FJ] Hypernephroma of the ovary. *British Medical Journal* 1921;2:531–2
[Unsigned, but Browne later cited himself as author of this 'critical review'].

1922
Ballantyne JW, Browne FJ. The problems of foetal post-maturity and prolongation of pregnancy. *Journal of Obstetrics and Gynaecology of the British Empire* 1922;29:177–238.

Browne FJ. Neo-natal death. *British Medical Journal* 1922;2:590–3.

Browne FJ. Pneumonia neonatorum. *British Medical Journal* 1922;1:469–71.

Miller J, Browne FJ. Extra-genital chorion-epitheliomata of congenital origin (with report of a new case of chorion-epithelioma in a male). *Journal of Obstetrics and Gynaecology of the British Empire* 1922;29:48–67.

1923
Browne FJ. On the influence of pregnancy on the Wassermann Reaction and on the clinical manifestations of syphilis. *Journal of Obstetrics and Gynaecology of the British Empire* 1923;30:519–40.

1924
Browne FJ. Further observations on still-birth and neonatal death: their causes, pathology and prevention. *Transactions of the Edinburgh Obstetrical Society* 1923–1924;XLIV:158–203.

Browne FJ. The induction of labour by quinine and pituitrin. *Transactions of the Edinburgh Obstetrical Society* 1923–1924;XLIV:25–33.
[For details of the extensive discussion following the presentation of this paper and a subsequent one by William Fordyce, see pages 36–42 and 47–53.]

1925

Browne FJ. On the abnormalities of the umbilical cord which may cause antenatal death. *Journal of Obstetrics and Gynaecology of the British Empire* 1925;32:17–48.

1926

Browne FJ. A case of concealed haemorrhage with placenta praevia. *Transactions of the Edinburgh Obstetrical Society* 1925–1926;XLVI:129–32.

Browne FJ. An experimental investigation into the etiology of accidental haemorrhage and placental infarction. *British Medical Journal* 1926;1:683–7.

Browne FJ. An experimental investigation into the etiology of accidental haemorrhage and placental infarction. *Transactions of the Edinburgh Obstetrical Society* 1925–1926;XLVI:151–68.

Browne FJ. The new obstetric unit. *University College Hospital Magazine* 1926;XI:210–18.

1927

Browne FJ. Venereal diseases in pregnancy. *British Medical Journal* 1927;2:250–3.

Blacker G, Browne FJ. University College Hospital: new obstetric hospital and residents' quarters. In: *Methods and Problems of Medical Education* 1927 8th series. p. 247–59.

1928

Browne FJ. A note on the immediate repair of the torn perineum under local anaesthesia *Lancet* 1928;1:1281.

Browne FJ. Some things of importance in obstetric practice *Medical World* 1928;XXVIII:222–8.

Browne FJ. The management of cases of venereal disease in ante-natal and post-natal clinics, and the arrangements for treatment. *Hospital Social Service* 1928;XVII:395–406.

Browne FJ, Dodds GH. Further experimental observations on the aetiology of accidental haemorrhage and placental infarction. *Journal of Obstetrics and Gynaecology of the British Empire* 1928;35:661–92.

1929
Browne FJ. Impressions of a visit to certain obstetrical and gynaecological clinics in the United States and Canada. *University College Hospital Magazine* 1929;XIV:215–37.

1930
Browne FJ. Correspondence. *University College Hospital Magazine* 1930;XV:163–70.
[Browne's response to an editorial, p. 57–61, concerning the work of the Obstetric Hospital and the introduction of antenatal care.]

Browne FJ, Dodds GH. Occult nephritis and its relation to pregnancy toxaemias. *Journal of Obstetrics and Gynaecology of the British Empire* 1930;37:476–82.

1931
Browne FJ. Sugar in the urine in pregnancy. *Medical World* 1931;XXXIV:437–41.

Browne FJ. A fatal case of acute puerperal inversion of the uterus. *Proceedings of the Royal Society of Medicine* 1931;24:1625–6.

Browne FJ. The value of the pregnancy reaction of Zondek and Ascheim in diagnosis and prognosis of chorion epithelioma. *Proceedings of the Royal Society of Medicine* 1931;24:1628–32.

Browne FJ. The health of the woman citizen as potential and actual mother. *Journal of State Medicine* 1931;39:688–702.

1932

Browne FJ. Antenatal care and maternal mortality. *Lancet* 1932;2:1–4.

Browne, FJ. High blood pressure as an early sign of toxaemia of pregnancy. *British Medical Journal* 1932;1:320–2.

1933

Browne FJ. The early signs of pre-eclamptic toxaemia, with special reference to the order of their appearance and their inter-relation. *Journal of Obstetrics and Gynaecology of the British Empire* 1933;40:1160–74.

1934

Browne FJ. Are we satisfied with the results of ante-natal care? *British Medical Journal* 1934;2:194–7.

Browne FJ. How can the results of ante-natal care be improved? *Proceedings of the Royal Society of Medicine* 1934;28:461–5.
[Browne's contribution to a joint Discussion of the Section of Epidemiology and State Medicine and the Section of Obstetrics and Gynaecology held on 23 November 1934. See p. 453–68 for the discussion in its entirety.]

1935

Browne FJ. Treatment of placenta praevia. *Lancet* 1935;2:959–61.

Browne FJ. Septic abortion and its treatment. *Medical Press and Circular* 1935;190: Supplement: Symposium No 1: Gynaecological emergencies, 1935:vi–xi.

1936

Browne FJ. Maternity services: the part played by education of medical students. *British Medical Journal* 1936;2:384–5.

Browne FJ. Antenatal care. In: *British Encyclopaedia of Medical Practice*, edited by Sir Humphry Rolleston. 1936, Volume 1, Butterworth, London, p. 601–20.
[Section 5, p. 617–620, entitled 'Antenatal care in the tropics' is contributed by VB Green-Armytage].

Browne FJ, Dodds GH. The cause of hypertension in pre-eclamptic toxaemia: a study of the blood pressure in mother and infant. *Lancet* 1936;1:1059–60.

1937

Browne FJ. The diagnosis and treatment of early malignant disease of the uterus. *Practitioner* 1937;138:11–23.

Browne FJ. Preventive medicine – 1: Antenatal care. *University College Hospital Magazine* 1937;XXII:169–76.

1938

Browne FJ. The staffing of ante-natal and child welfare clinics from the point of view of the obstetrician. *Journal of the Royal Institute of Public Health and Hygiene* 1937–1938;1:412–16.

Browne FJ. Placenta: development and diseases. In: *British Encyclopaedia of Medical Practice*, edited by Sir Humphry Rolleston. 1938, Volume 9, Butterworth, London, p. 641–74.

Browne FJ. Pregnancy: normal and pathological. *British Encyclopaedia of Medical Practice*, edited by Sir Humphry Rolleston. 1938 Volume 10, Butterworth, London, p. 48–125.

1939

Browne FJ. A criticism of current views on the value of Vitamin E in habitual abortion. *Proceedings of the Royal Society of Medicine* 1939;32:863–4.

Browne FJ. On the danger of Willett's forceps in placenta praevia with two illustrative cases. *Proceedings of the Royal Society of Medicine* 1939;32:1209–11.

Browne FJ, Dodds GH. The remote prognosis of the toxaemias of pregnancy: based on a follow-up study of 400 patients in 589 pregnancies for periods varying from 6 months to 12 years. *Journal of Obstetrics and Gynaecology of the British Empire* 1939;46:443–61.

1940

Browne FJ. The cold pressor test in pregnancy. *Journal of Obstetrics and Gynaecology of the British Empire* 1940;47:365–70.

Browne FJ, Dodds GH. The prognosis for the foetus in the toxaemias of late pregnancy. *Journal of Obstetrics and Gynaecology of the British Empire* 1940;47:549–52.

Dodds GH, Browne FJ. Chronic nephritis in pregnancy. *Proceedings of the Royal Society of Medicine* 1940;33:737–40.

1942

Browne FJ, Dodds GH. Pregnancy in the patient with chronic hypertension *Journal of Obstetrics and Gynaecology of the British Empire* 1942;49:1–17.

1943

Browne FJ. Reactions to pressor substances in normal and toxaemic women *Journal of Obstetrics and Gynaecology of the British Empire* 1943;50:254–9.

Browne FJ. Common ailments of pregnancy. *Mother and Child* 1943;14(6 September):135–8.

Browne FJ. On the value of vitamin B1 in prevention of toxaemia of pregnancy *British Medical Journal* 1943;1:445–6.

1944

Browne FJ. The significance of signs and symptoms in toxaemia of pregnancy. *Edinburgh Medical Journal* 1944 New Series;51:449–59. [Appears also in *Edinburgh Postgraduate Lectures in Medicine* 1948;4:124–34].

Browne FJ. Diet in pregnancy [Editorial commentary]. *British Encyclopaedia of Medical Practice. Medical Progress.* Edited by Sir Humphry Rolleston. Butterworth, London 1944 p. 144–5.

Browne FJ. The aetiology of the toxaemias of late pregnancy. *Journal of Obstetrics and Gynaecology of the British Empire* 1944;51:438–71.

1945

Barnes J, Browne FJ. Blood pressure and the incidence of hypertension in nulliparous and parous women in relation to the remote prognosis of the toxaemias of pregnancy. *Journal of Obstetrics and Gynaecology of the British Empire* 1945;52:1–12.

Barnes J, Browne FJ. Blood-pressure of relatives of patients with toxaemia of late pregnancy (a preliminary note). *Journal of Obstetrics and Gynaecology of the British Empire* 1945;52:559–69.

Browne FJ. La significacion y genesis de los signos y sintomas en la toxemia del embarazo. *Revista espanola de obstetricia y ginecologia* 1945;2:377–89. [Spanish translation of paper published in 1944 in the *Edinburgh Medical Journal.*]

1946

Browne FJ. Sensitization of the vascular system in pre-eclamptic toxaemia and eclampsia. *Journal of Obstetrics and Gynaecology of the British Empire* 1946;53:510–18.

Browne FJ. Obstetrics and gynaecology. In: *British Encyclopaedia of Medical Practice. Medical Progress.* Edited by Lord Horder. Butterworth, London, 1946, p. 21–9.

Browne FJ. Obstetrics and gynaecology. In: *British Encyclopaedia of Medical Practice. Medical Progress.* Edited by Lord Horder. Butterworth, London, 1947, p. 21–9.

Browne FJ. Obstetrics and gynaecology. In: *British Encyclopaedia of Medical Practice. Medical Progress.* Edited by Lord Horder. Butterworth, London, 1948, p. 28–36.

1947

Browne FJ. Antenatal and intranatal care. In: *Child health and development, by various authors.* Edited by Richard WB Ellis. Churchill, London, 1947, p. 15–38.

Browne FJ. Chronic hypertension and pregnancy. *British Medical Journal* 1947;2:283–7.

1949

Browne FJ. Chronic hypertension in pregnancy. In: *Transactions of the XIIth British Congress of Obstetrics and Gynaecology, held at Friends House, Euston Road, London NW1.* Edited by AW Bourne and WCW Nixon. Austral Press, on behalf of the Congress Committee, London, [1949], p. 143–58.

Browne FJ. Failed forceps. *British Medical Journal* 1949;2:975–6.

1950

Browne FJ. Observations on the origin of the lower uterine segment in pregnancy. *Proceedings of the Royal Society of Medicine* 1950;43:103–5.

1951

Browne FJ. Menorrhagia and metrorrhagia. In: *British Encyclopaedia of Medical Practice.* Edited by Lord Horder. Butterworth, London. 2nd ed. 1951, Volume 8, p. 488–501.

Browne FJ. Obstetrics and gynaecology. *University College Hospital Magazine* 1951;36:147–9.

1953

Browne FJ. Medical practice in Australia. *University College Hospital Magazine* 1953;XXXVIII (May, Coronation Number):17–21.

1955

Browne FJ. The National Health Service in Great Britain and its effect on the nursing profession. *Australian Nurses Journal* 1955;53:69–71, 80–3.

1956

Browne FJ, Sheumack DR. Chronic hypertension following pre-eclamptic toxaemia; the influence of familial hypertension on its causation. *Journal of Obstetrics and Gynaecology of the British Empire* 1956;63:677–9.

1957

Browne FJ. Maternal and foetal prognosis in toxaemias of pregnancy. *Medical Journal of Australia* 1957;44:198–200.

Browne FJ. Foetal post-maturity and prolongation of pregnancy. *British Medical Journal* 1957;1:851–5.

Browne FJ. A case of chorionepithelioma of the uterus with pulmonary metastases cured by operation and x-rays. *Journal of Obstetrics and Gynaecology of the British Empire* 1957;64:852–6.

1958

Browne FJ. Aetiology of pre–eclamptic toxaemia and eclampsia: fact and theory. *Lancet* 1958;1:115–20.

Browne FJ. The aetiology of pre–eclamptic toxaemia and eclampsia. *Bulletin of Post–Graduate Committee in Medicine, University of Sydney*, September 1958:250–51.
[Abbreviated text of *Lancet* article, January 1958].

Browne FJ. Toxaemias of pregnancy: a survey of the present position. *Nursing Mirror* 1958;30:v–vi.

Browne FJ. Standards on obstetrics. *Journal of Obstetrics and Gynaecology of the British Empire* 1958;65:826–31.

Reports

Browne FJ (1924) On the weight and length of normal foetuses and the weights of foetal organs, based on a series of 218 selected cases in Edinburgh. In: *Child life investigations: the estimation of foetal age, the weight and length of normal foetuses and the weights of foetal organs.* Medical Research Council, Special Report Series, No 86. HMSO, London, p. 65–87.

While working in Edinburgh, Browne submitted two reports to the Medical Research Council (MRC) on the subject of stillbirth. *Still birth: its causes, pathology and prevention,* May, 1921, was sent to Sir W Morley Fletcher on 14 June. The same recipient was notified on 16 November 1922 of the completion of a second report, *Further observations on still birth and neonatal death,* and Browne was instructed to send it direct to Dr Ballantyne for scrutiny. Neither report was published by the MRC but papers based upon these studies appeared from time to time in the medical press. Related correspondence has been deposited in The National Archives (TNA) by the MRC. [TNA Reference: FD 1/3892: *Dr FJ Browne's research, Edinburgh, 1920–1931*].

Also deposited in The National Archives are *Professor FJ Browne's and Miss FC Kelly's research on anaesthetics and obstetrics at University College Hospital, 1931–1935* [TNA Reference: FD 1/1678] and *Puerperal sepsis: research by Professor Browne and Professor Boycott, University College Hospital, London, 1929–1931* [TNA Reference: FD 1/2855].

Thesis

Browne FJ (1919) A contribution to the study of hydatidiform mole, with special reference to its association with lutein cysts of the ovary. MD Thesis, Aberdeen.

Index

Obstetrical Society of London
53
Obstetric Hospital (Unit),
University College Hospital
30–1, 32, 34–8, 46, 50
obstetrics 19, 42–3
development of 96–8
teaching 41–2, 44, 45
ovary, lutein cysts 17–18
Oxford University 28–9, 32

pain relief, in labour 37, 46–7
Peel, John 59, 71
pelvimetry, X-ray 33
Pembroke College, Cambridge
61, 73–4
Percival, Robert 54
perinatal mortality 96
pethidine 37, 46, 47
Philipp, Elliot 43, 80
Postgraduate Medical School,
Hammersmith 44, 70,
79–80
*Postgraduate Obstetrics and
Gynaecology* (FJ Browne)
44, 47, 70, 72, 80
postgraduate teaching 43–4,
79–80
postmaturity 23, 45, 54
postnatal clinics 31, 34
postpartum haemorrhage 28,
32, 45–6
pre-eclampsia *see* toxaemia of
pregnancy
Presbyterianism 41, 57, 81
Prince of Wales (later King
Edward VIII) 30
puerperal sepsis 34, 35

RANZCOG *see* Royal

Australian and New Zealand
College of Obstetricians and
Gynaecologists
Raphoe Royal School,
Donegal 5
Raymond, Mr 73
RCOG *see* Royal College of
Obstetricians and
Gynaecologists
Read, Charles 53, 72, 79–80
reading 59–60, 87
religion 41, 57
research 23–5, 33–4, 35–6, 38,
44–5
residents, medical 17, 19, 22,
30–1, 41, 42
Rickford, Braithwaite 54
Rivett, Carnac 54
Rockefeller Foundation 28–9,
35
Rodeck, Charles 34
Rosenheim, Max 32, 33, 36
Royal Academy of Music 71,
74
Royal Air Force (RAF) 62,
70, 73, 74
Royal Army Medical Corps
(RAMC) 8, 17
Royal Australian and New
Zealand College of
Obstetricians and
Gynaecologists
(RANZCOG)
archives 11, 12–13, 65, 82
FJ Browne medal 88–91
Royal College of Obstetricians
and Gynaecologists
(RCOG) 98
Fellowship (FRCOG)
51–2, 66

Printed in the United States
by Baker & Taylor Publisher Services

Printed in the United States
by Baker & Taylor Publisher Services